*Peak-
Performance
Living*

Also by Dr. Joel Robertson with Tom Monte

Natural Prozac

Peak-Performance Living

Dr. Joel C. Robertson
with Tom Monte

HarperSanFrancisco
An Imprint of HarperCollins*Publishers*

HarperSanFrancisco and the
authors, in association with the Basic
Foundation, a not-for-profit organization whose primary mission is refor-
estation, will facilitate the planting of
two trees for every one tree used in
the manufacture of this book.

A TREE CLAUSE BOOK

HarperCollins Web Site: http://www.harpercollins.com

HarperCollins®, ▄▄®, HarperSanFrancisco,™ and A TREE CLAUSE BOOK®
are trademarks of HarperCollins Publishers Inc.

FIRST HARPERCOLLINS PAPERBACK EDITION PUBLISHED
IN 1997
Set in Electra.

Library of Congress Cataloging-in-Publication Data

Robertson, Joel C.
Peak-performance living / Joel Robertson, with Tom Monte.

ISBN 0–06–251233–1 (cloth)
ISBN 0–06–251234–X (pbk.)
ISBN 0–06–251369–9 (intl. pbk.)

1. Neurochemistry.   2. Mood (Psychology).   3. Nutrition —
Psychological aspects.   4. Nutritionally induced diseases.
5. Health.   I. Monte, Tom.   II. Title.

QP356.3.R63   1996
612.8′042 — dc20   95–30971

97 98 99 00 01 ❖RRD(H) 10 9 8 7 6 5 4 3 2 1

Contents

Acknowledgments

As I began to complete this book, I realized the tremendous amount of energy and support many people have put into it. Whenever a book that has new and innovative information is published, a number of people must be involved to see the new vision carried out. This book is no exception. It is the result of not one or two individuals' efforts, but of several. The following people have been most influential in the process of completing this book.

First I would like to thank my wife, Vickie, and my three daughters, Nicole, Heidi, and Brooke, for their support and understanding while I researched and wrote this book. I couldn't have had the freedom to think and create without the support they have given me. They teach me more about what counts in this life than I can imagine. I love you gals.

I would also like to thank Tom Monte, an extraordinary writer, whose personality is evident throughout this book. His unique blend of emotional and intellectual processing was essential in making this book of practical use for readers. His tremendous efforts and talent have made it what it is. This truly is *our* book, not mine.

I would also like to thank my business associate, Brian Molitor, and his wife, Kathy, for their interest in and support of my family and our work.

To the people at Harper Collins Publishers. First to Tom Grady, vice president and publisher, for his continued vision for my work. Over the six years we have known each other, he has continued to encourage me to seek practical and informative solutions to people's needs. Caroline Pincus, a wonderful editor, whose insight and talent have polished this book. Robin Seaman, whose marketing skills are essential for a book like this to get to the audience that it is intended for. Cullen Curtiss and Sue White for their kindness, thoughtfulness, and efficiency in working out schedules and details, and keeping us all on track. Mary Peelen, a talented and creative publicist, for her patience and energy with deadlines. Emily Tilles, in publicity, for her involvement in the marketing of this book. Rosana Francescato, senior production editor, the detail person in making the manuscript accessible to the reader. And for all the others at Harper San Francisco—the sales team, office managers, and so on, who remained unnamed but not unappreciated. To the bookstore owners and managers for encouraging readers to read this book.

And finally, yet most important, to God, who provided the talent, that my family may share and try to make a difference in a world that is hard to understand.

Thank you to all.
Joel C. Robertson

Foreword

This book is the result of years of education and experience, as well as the observation of more than ten thousand people wishing to improve or change their lives. In my practice I have learned that just telling people what is best for them rarely brings about a change. In fact, most people know what they need to do long before they seek help; they are just unable to do it. For example, I have rarely met a person who was overweight or stressed or drank excess amounts of alcohol who didn't know what their problems were. But changing their behavior is difficult for most people. Contrary to my education, I concluded that such people aren't noncompliant and unwilling or unmotivated, but that the solutions professionals provide for them are inconsistent with their brain chemical reward system. In other words, they get no reward for their exercise programs, diets, or behavioral changes.

When I surveyed my peers and related professionals about their recommendations to people, I found they used generic or "one-size-fits-all" approaches. For example, one common recommendation is that everyone should exercise. But I asked the questions, what type of exercise, how long, how frequent? Should people exercise alone or with others? Before becoming stressed or to relieve stress they are already feeling? No one had answers to these questions. In essence, they didn't know how to tailor a program for patients, so instead they allowed patients to choose what felt good. I learned early in my career that what feels good—workaholism, gambling, drinking alcohol, using drugs—isn't always good. A better approach needs to be taken.

This book is the result of a new approach, the approach of self-care. Self-care starts with learning about your physiology—more specifically, your brain. This knowledge enables you to develop rewards from changing your behaviors, improving your thinking, and minimizing negative effects from adverse conditions. In this fashion, you—not your spouse, your children, your friends, your employer—make healthy choices about how to improve your performance.

The beginning of self-care is understanding the chemical rewards the brain provides when a person engages in certain behaviors or eats certain foods. Knowing how these rewards work will help you understand your spouse, friends, employer, and employees, as well as yourself.

Next you will learn about the behaviors, both positive and negative, you engage in without even thinking. I call them automatic behaviors. These behaviors frequently decrease your performance and efficiency.

Finally, you will learn about your personal brain chemistry. Do you have a chemical imbalance or is stress causing you to develop an imbalance? You can tailor specific diet, exercise, and behavior plans that you will stick to and enjoy, all the while improving your performance.

Learning about your personal brain chemistry will help you understand how your physiology drives you and your thinking process. For those of you interested in even more specific information, I have included at the back of this book a Performance Enhancement Survey, which can be returned to the Robertson Institute for a comprehensive report and suggestions for your enhancement.

The information in this book is exciting and the result of very interesting research. You will find it not only helpful but essential in your quest for peace and productivity. For the first time, you will be able to balance your understanding of psychological dynamics with an understanding of the physiology of your brain.

Enjoy reading and God Bless,
Joel C. Robertson

*Peak-
Performance
Living*

Introduction

Every day, whether we know it or not, we alter our brain chemistry. We do this through what we eat, what we do, and what we think. These changes in brain chemistry cause transformations in mood and intellectual performance that range from the subtle to the profound.

From time to time, by some accident of behavior and food selection, we manage to achieve a balanced brain chemistry, which triggers feelings of optimism, well-being, confidence, and intellectual clarity. For a day or two, we are imbued with a subtle joyousness. We have lots of energy. New ideas and insights spring to life, along with just the right words to express them. Mind and body are tuned and in perfect harmony. In short, we feel great.

All too quickly, however, the magic passes. We soon find ourselves fighting back irritability or anxiety, listlessness or depression. That all-too-familiar intellectual fog settles on us, and once again we're forgetting little things and fumbling for the right words. We feel uncomfortable physically and mentally, out of step with the rest of life. Ironically, we tend to accept these negative conditions as normal and regard the positive feelings as too good to last.

The fact is that we have much more power than we realize to shape our inner world. Because we are unaware of this power, however, most of us manage to manipulate our brain chemistry and our inner conditions to our own detriment. Yet we also have the ability to overcome these negative moods and stimulate a new round of positive feelings, inner strength, mental alertness, and hope. Most important, with awareness of our own power, we can *maintain* this peak-performance state.

To do this, we must realize that our daily behavior—including our food choices and the kinds of activities we engage in—helps to create our emotions, thoughts, and psychological states. We are capable of creating an enormous range of emotions and intellectual functioning. We can stimulate feelings of mild emotional discomfort, irritability, and intellectual fatigue; we can also give rise to real anxiety, fear, and depression. On the other hand, we can promote feelings of optimism, intellectual clarity, sharpened memory, and deep feelings of well-being. We can make it easier to enjoy deep and restful sleep. And we can even deal with many longstanding psychological and physiological conflicts that are rooted in brain chemistry imbalances. The degree of our discomfort or well-being depends on how close we are to a balanced neurochemistry.

Many people in our society reach for a drug when they want to alter their mood. But this is not only unhealthy, it's unnecessary. You can learn how to use behaviors and dietary choices to balance your neurochemistry and thus experience your best self.

That's the purpose of this book: to help you determine which foods and behaviors will help you feel better, perform better, and look better. As you will see, some of these positive changes can be accomplished quickly, often with a single meal or a specific activity. Others require consistent behavior, but even here results can come quickly. Knowing which foods and behaviors to adopt will promote feelings of well-being and positive emotions, enhance your performance at business meetings and presentations, and help you establish greater intimacy with loved ones. Most important, it will help you create long-term physical and psychological health.

The Road to Peak Performance

Over the past twenty years, I have treated more than ten thousand people for various kinds of emotional and psychological imbalances. In this process, I have learned that all of us use food and behavior to deal with stress and emotional pain, as well as to promote positive feelings and intellectual ability. Most of us manipulate our brain chemistry badly—we unwittingly engage in activities and eat foods that create neurochemical imbalances. These imbalances dull the mind, weaken the body, and cause needless emotional suffering. In the course of my work, I have developed a series of programs to show people how they can use behavior to promote positive feelings and enhanced intellectual abilities. I'm going to show you how you can increase your energy and intellectual clarity, improve your concentration, experience deeper sleep, and boost self-confidence and self-esteem. In short, I will describe a program that will help you achieve your peak performance.

I should stress that all of my methods are safe, natural, and scientifically proven. I use only food, nutrition, exercise, and a variety of mental and spiritual practices, all of which are designed to correct neurochemical imbalances that are currently causing a cacophony of desires, impulses, and emotional states. Once any of us achieves a balanced condition, our dark emotional clouds begin to dissipate. Meanwhile, our underlying abilities, talents, and unique characteristics can emerge.

The mechanism by which these changes occur is a delicate but powerful group of chemicals inside the brain called *neurotransmitters*. Neurotransmitters create a wide spectrum of feelings, moods, and thoughts—everything from depression, mania, anxiety, compulsivity, and addiction to feelings of self-confidence, self-esteem, clarity of thought, enhanced memory, healthy aggression, and deep sleep.

During the past twenty years, science has learned that neurotransmitters can be affected, often dramatically, by a wide variety of everyday behaviors. One of the most powerful—and fastest acting—is our food choices.

"It is becoming increasingly clear that brain chemistry and function can be influenced by a single meal," wrote Massachusetts Institute of Technology scientist John D. Fernstrom, Ph.D. "That is, in well-nourished individuals consuming normal amounts of food, short-term changes in food composition can rapidly affect brain function" (*Nutrition Action Newsletter,* December 1979).

Depending on our food choices, we can create any number of internal states. For example, foods rich in carbohydrates tend to boost levels of serotonin, a neurotransmitter that is responsible for giving you a feeling of well-being and goodwill. Serotonin increases your ability to concentrate on a particular subject or problem for extended periods of time. It also provides you with deeper and more restful sleep. When serotonin is high, people tend to be relaxed. They experience little or no anxiety or fear. When serotonin levels are low, depression is common; so is poor sleep and an inability to concentrate. Scientists at the University of California at Los Angeles and other research centers have shown that people who are chronically low in serotonin are often chronically depressed; some are prone to violence, against both others and themselves.

Another important neurotransmitter is dopamine, which has the opposite effects of serotonin. High levels of dopamine cause people to experience arousal, alertness, anxiety, and feelings of aggression. If dopamine remains abnormally high, anxiety can become severe— even to the point of paranoia, schizophrenia, and psychosis. Low dopamine can result in depression and disorders of the nervous and muscular systems. Like serotonin, dopamine levels rise and fall based upon the availability of certain nutrients and upon our daily behavior.

Diets rich in protein raise brain levels of dopamine and its related neurotransmitter, norepinephrine.

Serotonin and dopamine tend to have opposite effects on mood and behavior, and are often seen as the two chemicals that we are trying to balance to achieve a more harmonious emotional and psychological condition. Other neurochemicals play more subtle but equally important roles.

Food, however, is not the only influence on brain chemistry. Running, walking, stretching, singing, listening to music, watching television, gambling, overeating, praying, and sex are just a handful of the ways that we may alter our brain chemistry each day. In fact, all behavior has a corresponding chemical reaction in the brain that, in turn, changes us physiologically and psychologically.

What Are Automatic Behaviors?

Most of the behavior that has such a profound effect on your brain chemistry and your emotional and intellectual life is done unconsciously—you don't realize that you're doing it. Some of these *automatic behaviors* may be preventing you from reaching higher levels of your ability and emotional well-being.

Most of us function within a certain range of emotions and intellectual efficiency that do not approach our peak-performance capabilities. The reason we are unable to reach our potential is that we fill up our lives with negative thoughts, self-defeating behaviors, and foods that reinforce our neurochemical imbalances or make them worse. Consequently, we function under an extreme burden.

You may experience this as a sluggish or forgetful mind, excess aggression, too much passivity and too little willpower, or chronic anxiety or depression. Interestingly, you may be well aware that your mind is functioning a step or two slower than you would like; you may recognize that you're too aggressive or too passive. Indeed, some inner voice may be telling you that you are capable of living at a higher level of performance.

Many of these limitations are actually the effects of automatic behaviors. In this book you will learn more about the effects of your automatic behaviors and how you can change them.

Is It Okay to Change Our Brain Chemistry?

It's a strange side effect of our Puritanical society that most of us feel that it's okay to manipulate our brain chemistry *as long as we don't know that we're doing it.* The idea of *consciously* changing our behavior to make ourselves feel better makes some of us uncomfortable. Some worry about becoming robotic or computer-like. Others suffer from a kind of Promethean guilt about letting loose secrets that "rightly" belong to the unconscious or intuitive mind. Still others question whether, by consciously influencing our own brain chemistry, we aren't reprogramming ourselves. Have we finally entered Huxley's *Brave New World*?

The answer is an unequivocal *no*. First, every one of us should be questioning the adverse effects of modern life on the human organism—and especially on our brain's delicate chemistry and our own mental health. We should wonder whether the stresses of modern life, which are unlike any in previous human experience, aren't causing aberrations in neurochemistry and human behavior. Indeed, human beings have been progressively changed by eating certain types of foods and living in ways that naturally supported our physical, psychological, and spiritual well-being. Many of those foods and behaviors are foreign to us today.

As you know, the lifestyles of your grandparents and great-grandparents were a lot more physically demanding than our own. Also, your grandparents didn't eat the quantities of red meat, sugar, refined foods, and artificial ingredients that we do. They didn't experience the air, water, and soil pollution that burdens us. They didn't live isolated lives, and they didn't experience the same types of emotional and psychological stresses that we do. I could go on and on, and so could you. This is not to say that life in the past was ever easy. It wasn't. But it was more consistent with the human development and historical patterns than our current ways of living. Our modern world has made a break with those patterns, and therefore its effects on brain chemistry are more unpredictable.

Many scientists—and I am one of them—maintain that standard Western diet, our sedentary lifestyles, the pressures of time, and the continual bombardment of arousing stimuli (such as violent and sexual media images) all combine to create stresses on our neurochemistry that deform and distort our behavior. You are being pulled in so many directions that you hardly have the time or the peace to figure out who you are or what you really want to do in life. Little wonder, therefore, that our society suffers from so much drug and alcohol abuse, that our films and other media portray ever more graphic sex and violence. It's no wonder that many people today suffer from acute brain chemistry imbalances; the only way they know how to cope is with strong chemicals or extreme forms of behavior.

I'm not suggesting that we re-create the past. But we can combine the better aspects of our traditional wisdom with the profound insights of modern science to create lifestyles that will support our mental, emotional, and physical health. That's what I have done in the program described in this book. In another time and context, the food, nutrition, and behaviors used in my program would seem like common sense.

Brain, Mind, or Spirit?

Many people wonder if our efforts to balance brain chemistry ignore the presence of a higher consciousness or spirit within us. Actually, the brain-chemistry model demonstrates that a higher consciousness is what truly motivates changes in brain chemistry.

The brain is that mysterious matrix where the physical and the invisible mingle and become one. Here, nerve fibers and chemical messengers form the highway for the invisible realm of thoughts, emotions, mood states, memories, creativity, inspiration, beliefs, hopes, and dreams. Scientists, philosophers, and clergy have argued for centuries over which realm—the physical world of tissues and biochemistry or the invisible world of thoughts and spirit—serves as the origin of our humanity. Despite their seemingly irreconcilable differences, all sides agree that each of these realms dramatically alters the other. As science has proven, if we change the condition of the brain's neurons and chemistry, our thoughts and emotions change. The reverse is also true: change our thoughts and emotions, and the chemicals within our brains are also changed.

In a sense, the relationship between our emotions, thoughts, and psychological states and our neurons and brain chemistry can be seen as a chain of events that form a circle. Each link in the chain influences the next and makes the circle possible.

Nevertheless, when scientists confront the question of which is the higher authority, the brain or the mind-spirit, most agree that the mind-spirit is the higher center. That invisible part of you, the "I" that you recognize as your psychological and spiritual self, can profoundly alter your brain chemistry and function.

Nobel laureate Roger Sperry, whose pioneering work on the split-brain is one of the great breakthroughs in our understanding of this mysterious organ, says that our living consciousness—what most of us term the mind—is the commander of the brain. In *The Three Pound Universe*, by Judith Hooper and Dick Teresi, they say that ideas "call the plays, exerting downward control over the march of nerve-impulse traffic." Another Nobel Prize winner for discoveries of how the brain works, Sir John Eccles, has argued forthrightly that the human soul operates the brain, much like a person operates a computer. Whether you see it as the soul or the higher mind, the fact remains that something higher and invisible directs much of the brain's reactions. As one leading researcher put it, hope triggers the neurons to fire.

As I will show in later chapters, thoughts and ideas that are maintained consistently over time cause long-term changes in brain chemistry and function. We are shaped by what we think—especially if we think those thoughts consistently over a long enough period of time. One of the secrets to making long-term changes in brain chemistry is through consistent types of thinking—optimism, for example, or faith. Certain daily practices, such as meditation, prayer, and relaxation exercises, can foster these long-term, positive changes in brain chemistry.

Most of us find it easier to think positively and use the powers of our minds after we've reduced or eliminated other toxic influences in daily life. I encourage you to begin with changes in food choices, and to move on to change daily behaviors. Once you begin to use these tools, your change in mood and performance will quickly tell you that transformation has already begun.

Terri's Story

As a short illustration of how the program works, let me tell you about Terri, a thirty-two-year-old woman with a history of compulsive overeating, depression, and control issues. Terri had tried every diet imaginable to control her weight, without any kind of enduring success. Whenever she adopted a new program, she'd lose weight; but within a few months the pounds would be back—and then some. Interestingly, when Terri adopted a new diet, she became exceedingly compulsive about the details of the program. That compulsivity extended to other areas of her life, including an increased need to control her husband's behavior. After several attempts at losing weight, Terri and her husband concluded that Terri was better off eating anything she wanted and being heavy, simply because she made life miserable for both of them when she was on a diet.

Terri heard about my program and came to me for help. First, I gave her a neurochemical evaluation. That's a series of tests I use to determine which of a small group of brain chemicals is imbalanced—

either too low or too high relative to the other neurochemicals. In Terri's case, her serotonin levels—levels of the neurotransmitter that enhances our ability to concentrate, enjoy deep sleep, and experience a sense of well-being—were exceedingly low. Other neurotransmitters, including dopamine—which increases anxiety and fears—were too high. We later determined that Terri's imbalance was caused by her lifestyle and diet, which contained few carbohydrates and large amounts of high-protein foods. The resulting imbalance made Terri both depressed and anxious, a combination that caused her to lose hope yet indulge in a wide array of compulsive behaviors.

I gave Terri a diet and behavioral plan that would boost her serotonin levels and thereby give her an increased sense of security, well-being, and improved concentration. The program had a dramatic and positive effect. Almost immediately, Terri's compulsivity decreased, which meant that she didn't need to obsess over my program as she had over others. Meanwhile, other emotional and psychological characteristics related to increased serotonin levels began to emerge. She felt safer, more relaxed, and better able to concentrate. Within six months, she had lost a significant amount of weight and was keeping it off—without being on a weight-loss program. This alone increased her self-esteem, but Terri's emotional and physical health were also enhanced by the program. She was no longer chronically depressed. On the contrary, she noticed that her occasional downward turns of emotion were short-lived and passing, more like a cloud floating before the sun. Her bright outlook returned quickly. At the same time, she became much more flexible and open in her life.

Terri is a good example of how life stabilizes when we reduce or eliminate automatic behaviors that cause us so much pain.

Your Program for Peak Performance

I have designed a series of self-tests that will help you identify which, if any, of your neurotransmitters are currently imbalanced. By answering the questionnaires, you'll be able to understand which brain chemicals are excessive and which ones may be deficient. In this way, you'll come to know the causes of your slow or rapid mental functioning (whichever the case may be), as well as the causes of erratic mood swings, chronic anxiety, depression, or any compulsive behaviors you may have. Once you understand the specific imbalance, you can adopt a program that's appropriate to your particular condition.

In my work with over ten thousand patients, I have seen that certain neurochemical imbalances give rise to certain characteristics and even specific personality types. This stands to reason, since those who are excessive in, say, dopamine are likely to be more aggressive than those who are deficient in dopamine, just as those who have normal serotonin levels will experience greater inner peace than those who are low in serotonin.

I have divided the most general kinds of neurochemical imbalances into two separate and distinct personality types, which I call the Arousal personality and the Satiation personality. Virtually everyone alive falls into one of these two general categories. As you begin to understand the neurochemical model and answer the questionnaires, you will see clearly which type you are. Later, we will divide these general categories into 4 types—two Satiation personalities and two Arousal personalities—and offer appropriate diet and exercise programs for each.

You can gain an even deeper understanding of your neurochemistry and your personality by reading chapters 9 to 18, which explain the nine neurochemical types—four Satiation, four Arousal, and one combined type. A series of self-tests will help you recognize which of the nine types you are, and how to tailor your diet and exercise program to achieve neurochemical balance for your type.

In this book, we are going to explore how behavior affects our brain's chemistry and how we can achieve peak performance and optimal health. But as you will soon find out, there are no ironclad formulas within these pages, and nothing here to turn you into a robot or a super-human. Rather, you will find tools to improve your moods, sharpen your mental faculties, and help you function more effectively in specific situations. This book will also help you make the wisest choices possible so that you can make short- and long-term positive changes in your physical, mental, and emotional life.

1

The Biology of Moods and Performance

Understanding the Gas-Pedal and Brake-Pedal Chemicals

Good and bad moods, mental lethargy and states of anxiety and well-being, excitement, sexual arousal, and love seem to come and go like the weather—unpredictably and mysteriously. But our moods are not really as capricious as the weather. Moods, good and bad, arise in large part from electrical and chemical events inside our brains. Before we can begin to influence our moods toward balance, we need to understand how these biological events work.

The Body Electric

You may not think of yourself as being powered by electricity, but that is a big part of what makes the body work. Everything you touch, see, smell, hear, and taste is turned into electrical signals that speed through your nerves and to your brain. In fact, everything that you think about, experience as an emotion, or sense intuitively is converted into an electrical signal, and these signals are in turn converted to specific types of *neurochemicals*—chemicals in your brain. The type of chemical each signal produces depends on the kind of information it receives—from the tip of your finger or tongue, the type of food you just ate, or the kind of thought you just had. In short, experience—whether it is physical, emotional, intellectual, or spiritual—translates into electrical and chemical events that shape your inner world.

All of these events take place within tiny cells called *neurons*, the brain's basic unit. A neuron is shaped something like a star, with several short radiant arms, called *dendrites*, and one exceedingly long one, called an *axon*. The dendrites and axon spring from a cell body, in which lies the cell's nucleus and its cytoplasm.

Although thoughts seem to fire across the brain with lightning-like quickness, the actual process is more like a bucket-brigade, with one neuron passing information on to the next. It happens like this: A neuron fires an electrical charge from its cell body. The charge flies down the runway of an axon at a couple of hundred miles per hour until it reaches the axon's tip. There the charge stimulates the production of a *neurotransmitter*, a chemical that collects on the tip of the axon and then drips onto the adjoining neuron. The intensity of the charge that travels down the axon determines the effect of the wide variety of neurotransmitters the axon will release.

The neurotransmitter is caught by a *recepto*r specifically designed for that neurochemical and located on one of the dendrites of the adjacent neuron. When the neurotransmitter binds with the appropriate receptor, the information is passed from the dendrite to the cell body.

The type of neurotransmitter received tells the neuron what type of action to take, and what type of charge and chemical to pass on to the next neuron.

The result is the beautifully orchestrated physical, mental, and emotional reactions of the human body. Muscle cells in the finger may contract rhythmically to produce music; the brain may be informed of pain in the foot or burning at the fingers; hope is inspired by sudden news; sexual desire is aroused by an attractive partner; hunger or thirst is stimulated by the sight of food and drink. When things go wrong, however, any number of physical or mental disorders can arise, including stress, anxiety, depression, even schizophrenia and psychosis.

There's a tiny gap between neurons, called a *synaptic cleft*, where neurotransmitters make their jump from one neuron to the next. Here, in the synapse, are untold numbers of possibilities: so much can happen in that little leap that the neurotransmitter makes. It can be an all-or-nothing gambit—the neurotransmitter either clears the jump or doesn't, which means that the chain of events leading to a thought, a memory, or a specific action may be interrupted or never occur at all. Another possibility is that the presence of enzymes on the receptor of the neighboring neuron prevents the full effects of the neurotransmitter from being felt. When the neurochemical serotonin is low, for example, we may feel depressed. When acetylcholine is low, we may experience memory loss.

All the drugs that affect our thinking, emotions, and behavior have their greatest impact here, at the synapse. Drugs—including alcohol, caffeine, antidepressants, marijuana, and LSD—create changes at the synapse, thus creating significant alterations in the function of specific neurotransmitters. The response depends on the drug used. Each neurotransmitter has its own effect; when you increase the quantity of that chemical, you get an altered response, either heightened or depressed.

There are billions and billions of neurons in the brain. Some scientists believe there are 10 billion, others say there are 100 billion;

nobody knows for sure. Many of them die out naturally as we grow older; others are destroyed by alcohol or drug abuse. In any case, human development has seen to it that we have an overabundance of neurons, and usually only injury, illness, or addiction to alcohol or drugs will cause significant impairment of the brain.

Neurotransmitters: The Brain's Gas Pedals and Brake Pedals

Neurotransmitters have been called hormones or hormonelike substances because they set in motion specific functions within the body and nervous system, especially the brain. However, while some neurotransmitters trigger reactions, others slow reactions down. Thus neurotransmitters can be classified as either *excitatory* or *inhibitory*. The exciter neurotransmitters increase neurotransmission—that is, they speed up the transmission of a neurotransmitter from one neuron to another. The inhibitors slow down or weaken neurotransmission. I like to refer to the excitatory neurotransmitters as "gas pedals" and the inhibitors as "brake pedals."

Often, the gas-pedal and brake-pedal chemicals work together to modulate and coordinate movements. A good example of this is the combination of dopamine and acetylcholine. Dopamine is an excitatory neurotransmitter—it stimulates the muscles to contract. Acetylcholine, which in this case acts as an inhibitor, controls the rate of contraction and activity within the muscles. When the two are combined in perfect balance, muscles move in smooth, graceful harmony. Whether you tilt your head, walk down the street, play basketball or golf, or cook dinner, dopamine and acetylcholine are combining to coordinate your every move.

Problems arise when the two neurochemicals are not working together. This is precisely what happens in Parkinson's disease. Here, certain parts of the nervous system, located in a part of the brain called the basal ganglia, degenerate and are no longer able to produce adequate quantities of dopamine. As a result, acetylcholine acts as an inhibitor and dominates the information pathways within the nervous system and causes overly tense muscles, jerky movement, tremor, and the head shaking. In essence, the gas-pedal neurotransmitter is weak or inadequate, while the brake-pedal chemical is dominant. The result is tentative, uncertain, and inhibited movements.

Appropriate amounts of gas-pedal and brake-pedal chemicals play a role in many other essential activities that we take for granted. Memory, speech, the ability to sleep deeply and react to situations immediately all depend on having a balance between the excitatory and the inhibitor chemicals. When one or more of a single category becomes excessive, the effects are not only visible, but downright frustrating.

As we will see in a later chapter, the speed of neurotransmission is affected by the available energy within the cell, which is determined by the presence of an enzyme called *adenylate cyclase*. This enzyme converts potential or stored energy into usable or kinetic energy.

Our brains use more than a dozen neurotransmitters, but five of them appear to be both especially powerful and easily manipulated by our daily behaviors—and these are the ones we'll be discussing in this book. These five are acetylcholine, dopamine, gamma-aminobutyric acid (also known as GABA), norepinephrine, and serotonin; dopamine and serotonin especially seem to play a leading role in the play of our emotions and intellectual capabilities. All five are boosted or decreased by a number of factors in our daily lives, the most powerful of which are diet, exercise habits, beliefs, consistent thoughts, and behaviors. Let's look at all five of the neurotransmitters and the ways in which they are influenced by our daily behavior.

Dopamine: The Body's Rocket Fuel

Dopamine is an excitatory neurotransmitter. It is used by the brain to stimulate heightened states of alertness, awareness, and aggression. Dopamine accelerates transmission of nerve impulses from one neuron to the next, speeding up brain function and enhancing our ability to solve problems. When dopamine is elevated, we think, speak, and breathe more rapidly. Dopamine is also essential for all coordinated muscle movement.

Dopamine is used as a building block in the creation of norepinephrine, which is further converted to adrenaline. Dopamine, norepinephrine, and adrenaline are all involved in the familiar "fight-or-flight" reactions of the brain and body. All responses involving fear—increased cardiovascular, respiratory, and muscle activity—depend on heightened levels of dopamine and norepinephrine. Not surprisingly, balanced levels of dopamine are essential for healthy perceptions of reality.

When mildly elevated, dopamine increases:

- arousal
- awareness and alertness
- assertiveness
- aggression
- respiration, cardiovascular, and muscle activity

Moderately elevated dopamine levels can lead to:

- anxiety (consistent elevations can lead to chronic anxiety)
- fear
- feelings of detachment
- sleep disturbances
- increased sex drive

Excessive dopamine that remains chronically high can lead to delusions, hallucinations, inappropriate responses and affect, paranoia, social isolation, withdrawal, schizophrenia, and psychosis.

Medications such as Haldol are used to block the effects of dopamine, and thus reduce the above-mentioned symptoms. Cocaine, on the other hand, temporarily increases production of dopamine, resulting in bursts of energy, euphoria, delusional thinking, paranoia, and fears. Ironically, cocaine—like other substances that cause extreme reactions in brain chemistry—eventually causes the opposite effect by depleting dopamine levels in the brain.

Low dopamine levels can cause:

- depression
- low energy
- muscular disturbances and Parkinson's disease
- the need for excess sleep
- withdrawal
- suicide or preoccupation with thoughts of suicide

Cocaine withdrawal causes low dopamine levels and results in extremes of these same symptoms, especially depression, withdrawal, sleep, and a craving for more cocaine (to return dopamine levels to normal).

Interestingly, recent research suggests that the overconsumption of animal proteins may be implicated in Parkinson's disease. Those who suffer from Parkinson's disease are usually given the medication L-dopa, which is used to produce dopamine in the brain. Scientists have discovered that L-dopa is more effective for those on high-carbohydrate, low-protein diets. Later in this book we'll be exploring diet, exercise, and lifestyle techniques to increase or lower dopamine levels.

Foods That Raise Dopamine Levels

The body uses the amino acid *tyrosine*, found in all protein foods, to produce dopamine. All protein-rich foods contain tyrosine, which will boost dopamine levels. Eating approximately three to four ounces of protein-rich food will elevate dopamine levels and have significant effects on mood and brain function. (See chapter 6 for information on the protein and fat content of individual foods.) Moreover, those effects occur rapidly, usually within thirty minutes of consumption of the protein food, and often in less than ten minutes.

Among the most protein-rich foods are:

- Fish: cod, haddock, flounder, scrod, halibut, fluke, salmon, sturgeon, sea bass, shark, tuna, mackerel, swordfish, and others.
- Poultry: chicken (preferably without the skin, which is where most of the fat is located), turkey, and eggs.
- Red meat: beef, lamb, veal, and pork.
- Beans: chickpeas, lentils, black beans, navy beans, pinto beans, soybeans, black-eyed peas, green beans.

How Exercise Affects Dopamine

Vigorous aerobic exercise utilizes available dopamine and thus temporarily depletes dopamine from the brain. This provides short-term relaxation to people with high levels of dopamine—*as long as the exercise is not a competitive sport.*

Competitive sports of any type *raise* dopamine levels and can keep them elevated well after the game has finished. In fact, all forms of competition—even common board games—can raise dopamine levels, as every chess player has experienced at one time or another. Competition triggers the survival instinct and fight-or-flight responses, signaling the production of dopamine, norepinephrine, and adrenaline. In the process, it increases anxiety, alertness, aggression, and fear. These biochemical events take place during the competition itself, but linger long after it, especially if you hate to lose and tend to berate yourself after losing.

Strenuous daily aerobic exercise *temporarily* depletes dopamine and thus provides relaxation to people with high dopamine. Noncompetitive exercises, such as running, stairmaster, skipping rope, cross-country skiing, and mountain biking, burn up dopamine and also raise serotonin levels somewhat. But the net effect of such exercise is to signal the body to produce more dopamine to replace lost stores of the excitatory neurochemical. The mechanisms are similar to the way exercise builds up muscle and bone. Initially, exercise breaks down muscle and bone tissue; this tells the body to produce more muscle and bone tissues, which makes both bigger, stronger, and better able to perform more work.

Dopamine replacement works in the same way. By burning up our stores of dopamine, the body is stimulated to produce more dopamine over time. Once dopamine increases, anxiety is elevated and we want to get back in the gym, do our exercises, and feel relaxed and sated once again. Yet, in time, the dopamine rises and keeps the cycle going.

In this way, exercise can easily become addictive — indeed, it does become an addiction for many long-distance runners and workout fanatics. These people feel bad when they are unable to get their regular workout, and that can be a problem. The symptoms they experience are specific to high dopamine: anxiety, stress, increased aggression, irritability, and inability to relax.

The best approach for some people with high dopamine is to mix up the exercise routine to include both highly demanding aerobic exercise and less demanding walking or stretching. The highly aerobic exercise will burn up dopamine and raise serotonin levels. Meanwhile, the mild aerobic exercise, such as walking or stretching, will boost serotonin. This combination will balance brain chemistry.

How Thoughts and Beliefs Affect Dopamine

All thoughts and images of excitement, activity, risk-taking, challenges, deadlines, gambling, sex, fear, anxiety, frightening scenarios, and beliefs that the future will present difficulties promote dopamine release. Simply thinking about taking a test, riding a roller-coaster, facing recrimination, fantasizing about sex, or conjuring up images in which you will be threatened — all of these and more promote the production and release of dopamine.

Clearly, then, our underlying psychology — our basic belief system — will determine our baseline chemistry to a great extent. That belief system also sets us up for all kinds of automatic behaviors or even addictions, because if we believe that we live under some sort of threat, our dopamine levels will be constantly up. Changing that baseline requires consistent behavior change, using diet, exercise, and thoughts that support the diminution of dopamine and the elevation of serotonin. Most of this book is directed at doing exactly that.

Serotonin: The Neurotransmitter of Inner Peace

We may think of self-esteem, confidence, or the ability to concentrate as invisible characteristics, grounded in the equally invisible psyche, but they too have roots in biochemistry. The neurotransmitter that corresponds with these and other positive traits is serotonin.

Serotonin is responsible for creating feelings of well-being, personal security, relaxation, and deep and restful sleep. Serotonin causes the brain to be less distracted and more focused, thus improving concentration. Studies at the Massachusetts Institute of Technology (MIT) and elsewhere have established that serotonin plays a role in pain relief and in reducing sensitivity to pain. Serotonin affects our perceptions dramatically. All balanced emotional conditions and even such elevated states as happiness and joy are associated with normal or high serotonin levels. On the other hand, insecurity, anger, fear, paranoia, depression, and even suicide are associated with low serotonin.

Both human and animal studies have shown that violence tends to manifest more frequently in men and animals with consistently low serotonin levels. Research done by the National Institutes of Mental Health (NIMH) on a group of military men revealed that those men who had the lowest levels of serotonin also had histories of antisocial behavior and far greater violence than those with higher serotonin levels. The researchers discovered that even among the violent men, those with the lowest levels of serotonin were prone to the greater violence.

Researchers at NIMH speculate that violence associated with low serotonin is ultimately turned inward, against oneself. Studies have shown that men who commit suicide, especially by violent acts, also tend to be low in serotonin.

Animal studies have confirmed many of the same human findings. Research on monkeys has demonstrated that those animals that are high in serotonin, and therefore less prone to violence, tend to be the leaders of the social network. One might think that it would be just the opposite: that the more violent animals would lead, since they would strike the most fear in the group. But no, the leaders tend to be more self-assured and balanced, and may exhibit less fear and insecurity than the others in the group. These characteristics are all associated with higher brain levels of serotonin.

In another series of studies, NIMH scientists have discovered that the depression associated with the lack of sunlight in winter is caused by a deficiency of serotonin. Seasonal Affective Disorder (known by the acronym SAD) occurs when the body produces high levels of a hormone called melatonin, which consumes serotonin. Melatonin is produced by the pineal gland, a small gland in the brain that is highly sensitive to light. The production of melatonin is suppressed by sunlight, but increases in many people who are deprived of adequate natural light, which often occurs in winter. Thus the higher the melatonin levels, the lower the serotonin levels, and the higher the rates of depression. Interestingly, MIT scientists have discovered that when serotonin levels decline (including in people with SAD), the body automatically craves carbohydrates, a nutrient that boosts serotonin.

People with low serotonin levels experience:

- declines in mood
- depression
- low energy and fatigue
- low self-esteem
- poor concentration
- difficulty making decisions

- fluctuations in appetite (usually manifesting as cravings for car-bohydrates, but little appetite for other foods)
- decrease in sex drive
- excessive feelings of guilt and unworthiness
- consistently low serotonin, which, as we have already seen, can lead to violence, antisocial behavior, and even suicide

What Causes High Levels of Serotonin?

Levels of serotonin far above normal usually do not occur naturally. Medications, such as the antidepressant Prozac, work by elevating serotonin levels. Antidepressants reduce and sometimes eliminate the negative symptoms associated with low serotonin. For some people, drugs such as Prozac create feelings of high self-esteem, confidence, the desire to express oneself, and the ability to bring out previously un-known abilities. For many who take such drugs, however, there are side effects that eventually require a cessation of the medication. The side effects often include anxiety, nervous tension, insomnia, drowsi-ness, tremors, sweating, gastrointestinal distress, nausea, diarrhea, diz-ziness, and lightheadedness.

Studies have shown that we can boost serotonin naturally with carbohydrate-rich diets, the kinds of exercises described above, medi-tation, and prayer. Inspiring music has been shown to elevate endor-phins, and may raise serotonin levels.

How Food Affects Serotonin Levels

Serotonin levels are increased by carbohydrates and carbohydrate-rich foods, all of which boost blood levels of *tryptophan,* an amino acid that acts as a precursor to serotonin. Although red meat and foods rich in animal proteins contain tryptophan, paradoxically serotonin levels go down when animal proteins are eaten.

This occurs because entry into the brain is guarded by the so-called blood-brain barrier. In order for amino acids to pass through the barrier, they must get onto a kind of transport system that restricts the number and kinds of amino acids that are allowed entry into the brain. Animal proteins are loaded with a wide array of amino acids, and they all compete for seats on the transport system. The net effect is that less tryptophan gets into the brain, and consequently less serotonin is produced.

This does not occur when carbohydrates are consumed, because the amount of tryptophan is greater relative to the amounts of other amino acids. Thus far more tryptophan gets into the brain and more serotonin is produced.

Foods that are rich in carbohydrates and therefore boost serotonin are:

- whole grains, such as brown rice, wheat, barley, oats, millet, corn, and buckwheat
- grain flour products, such as bread, pasta, rolls, crackers, bagels, cornbread, tortillas, chapati, and burritos
- sweet rolls and pastries, cookies, and other sweet flour foods
- carbohydrate-rich vegetables, such as potatoes, yams, sweet potatoes, and squashes
- simple sugar

All of these foods will boost serotonin levels—and quickly. About one-and-a-half ounces of carbohydrate food—a slice or two of bread, or a couple of cookies—will significantly boost brain levels of serotonin.

Fruit is loaded with carbohydrates, but not the kind that will directly affect your brain chemistry. The sugar found in fruit is mostly *fructose*, which must be broken down by enzymes in the small intestine before it can be converted to blood sugar, or *glucose*. This process, however, takes a considerable amount of time, which means that fruit is essentially a neutral agent on blood chemistry until its sugar is converted.

Fruit, however, is loaded with immune-boosting and cancer-fighting nutrients, such as the antioxidant vitamins C and A; it also contains fiber, which improves digestion. Fruit is a very healthy food and an essential part of a healthy diet.

How Exercise Affects Serotonin

Strolling in the park, walking in nature, bicycle riding on a flat surface, stretching exercises, reading, and prayer all promote the production of serotonin. The feelings that emerge whenever you walk in such places are profoundly quieting, meditative, and life-supportive. These experiences and the underlying feelings promote the production of serotonin. At the same time, your inner emotional state is elevated by the increasing levels of serotonin that are flooding your brain. Thus you have set up a positive cycle in which the exercise is producing serotonin, and the serotonin is boosting your mood.

All meditative exercise, such as stretching and low-impact aerobics, also boosts serotonin and thus promotes feelings of well-being, concentration, and inner peace. Prayer and meditation alone can also be serotonin boosters.

Acetylcholine: Muscles and Memory

Acetylcholine can serve as either an inhibitor or an excitatory neurotransmitter, depending on the presence and quantity of other neurotransmitters at the synapse.

Acetylcholine plays an essential role in smooth, coordinated muscle movements (including those of the heart) and in memory. Scientists have discovered that low levels of acetylcholine are associated with memory loss, Alzheimer's disease, and tardive dyskinesia, a disorder characterized by uncontrollable jerking movements of the face, tongue, and upper body.

Research has shown that when the amino acid choline is consumed (it is abundant in soybeans and eggs), acetylcholine is increased in the brain. Some patients with Alzheimer's disease who are fed high levels of choline show a slowing of the progression of the disease as compared to patients who are not given the choline. At least one study has shown that a minority of Alzheimer's patients fed high quantities of choline show an improvement in their symptoms. Other studies have failed to confirm this finding, however. Choline-rich foods may play a role in the prevention of Alzheimer's disease and other disorders associated with a deficiency of acetylcholine.

Low levels of acetylcholine result in difficulty with both short- and long-term memory, as well as decreased sex drive. Exceedingly low acetylcholine levels that do not manifest as Alzheimer's disease or other disorders are usually brought about by medications that block choline's effectiveness as the neurotransmitter's precursor.

People with low acetylcholine levels experience:

- impairment of vision (usually blurred vision)
- decreased sweating
- urine retention
- increased heart rate
- pounding heart
- loss of taste
- nervousness
- weakness
- drowsiness
- mental confusion
- impotence
- insomnia
- constipation

Because acetylcholine is usually an inhibitor, low levels enhance the other neurotransmitters that are dominant. Thus deficient acetylcholine may be unable to put the brake pedal on excess dopamine, causing elevated symptoms associated with too much of this gas-pedal neurotransmitter.

The symptoms of excess acetylcholine, usually caused by medication, include:

- excessive salivation
- vomiting
- uncontrollable urination and defecation
- sweating
- headache
- impairment of vision
- muscular weakness
- mania and manic behavior

Norepinephrine: Speeding Up Your Thoughts

Norepinephrine is another excitatory neurotransmitter. It is essential in all functions associated with heightened alertness, muscle activity, the constriction and dilation of blood vessels, elevated heart rate, and the opening of bronchioles in the respiratory tract.

Normal norepinephrine levels provide us with the ability to react quickly and aggressively to demanding situations and danger. It also protects us against depression that often is associated with the lack of will to take on projects or challenges. Norepinephrine increases the speed of your thoughts, or what I call *neurotransmission*. People with normal to high norepinephrine think and express themselves rapidly. (See chapter 5 for more on neurotransmission speed and norepinephrine.)

Norepinephrine Levels

Like dopamine, which is its precursor, norepinephrine is elevated by the consumption of protein-rich foods and, specifically, tyrosine, an amino acid that is abundant in fish, all forms of red meat, eggs, and low-fat dairy products.

The symptoms of low norepinephrine levels include:

- low energy
- depression
- weight gain
- changes in menstruation
- decreased sex drive

Chronically low norepinephrine can manifest as:

- attention deficit disorders
- obesity
- insomnia
- fatigue
- disorientation
- short-term memory loss
- dull or slow thought processes
- male impotence

Interestingly, the depression associated with low norepinephrine is much more vegetative than the depression associated with low serotonin. The reason is that low serotonin is often accompanied by relatively higher levels of dopamine and norepinephrine, both gas-pedal neurotransmitters. The result is depression accompanied by anxiety and fear, emotional states that usually create activity. Low norepinephrine levels, on the other hand, are often associated with low dopamine, which means that the depression has little of the fight or fear that normally accompanies the low serotonin depression. Thus the person sits in a kind of vegetative state, not caring what happens, one way or the other.

High levels of norepinephrine usually manifest as:

- anxiety
- excess energy

- racing and pounding heart
- increase in blood pressure
- decrease in insulin release
- increased breathing
- weight loss
- increased sex drive

The use of drugs that increase norepinephrine (most notably the antidepressant monoamine oxidase inhibitors, such as Nardil) often result in weight loss, anxiety, and phobias.

Gamma-Aminobutyric Acid (GABA): The Brain's Brake Pedal

Gamma-aminobutyric acid (GABA) is present in large quantities throughout the body. GABA plays a role in the modulation or lessening of anxiety. According to research done at the University of Pittsburgh, deficiencies of GABA have been found to be associated with increased anxiety and tension. Alcohol is known to increase GABA at the neuron receptor sites, and so relieves tension temporarily. Research has suggested that the sons of alcoholic fathers have lower levels of GABA, which makes them predisposed to needing alcohol to increase GABA, which in turn relieves tension and anxiety.

Interestingly, Valium, a mood-altering drug used to decrease anxiety, increases the action of GABA. This suggests that extremely low levels of GABA may also be associated with anxiety.

Symptoms of low GABA levels include:

- increased anxiety
- sleeplessness
- seizures

Symptoms of high GABA levels include:

- muscle relaxation
- quieting effects
- increased sleep

We each prefer to feel a certain way, according to our own inner nature. That inner you is grounded in your own unique neurochemical balance. In order to sustain that balance, your brain rewards you for certain behaviors, thus reinforcing who you are and how you like to feel. It is this reinforcement that may cause you trouble: Like most people, you may use foods and behaviors that provide short-term rewards but give you long-term problems. In order to get both the short- and long-term rewards (and keep them coming), you have to understand yourself a little better. For that deeper understanding, let's turn to chapter 2.

2

Understanding Your Baseline Emotional Tone

You Are Not Your Moods

Thelma was thirty-eight years old when she came to me complaining of the chronic depression that had plagued her for most of her life. Though she suffered only periodic bouts of deep depression, Thelma's general temperament was depressed and fatigued. She told me that her mother also experienced long periods of depression. Sometimes she slept all day, and complained of being just plain run down. With a little probing from me, Thelma recalled that her grandmother had complained of the same problem—chronic depression and fatigue.

Because such feelings were so much a part of her life and of her family's life, Thelma regarded depression as *familiar* and even *normal*.

Depression was part of what it meant to be Thelma, at least as far as Thelma was concerned. She never really expected to feel better; and perhaps on a much deeper level, she was a little afraid of feeling better because it meant feeling different. Depression was the background music that was constantly playing in Thelma's life: her baseline emotional tone.

A neurochemical evaluation (see the Performance Enhancement Survey at the back of this book) showed that Thelma had low serotonin levels. Occasionally, Thelma's job became stressful, which would drive up her brain levels of dopamine, triggering nervous tension, anxiety, and fear—feelings that Thelma regarded as unbearable. She'd rather be depressed—at least she knew what to expect. Whenever Thelma got stressed, she automatically withdrew not only from the stressor, but from much of life. Withdrawal caused her dopamine levels to fall, but it did little or nothing for her low serotonin. Consequently, Thelma went back to being depressed, though she had successfully lowered her anxiety. She had won a half-victory, and that was all she ever really expected out of life.

Thelma's experience typifies what a lot of us feel about coping with our moods. Though we may succeed in lessening the pain, we don't really expect to feel *good*. From the perspective of our lowered expectations, escape from acute pain is about as much of a victory as we can expect. Many who engage in such tactics believe, down deep, that life is a no-win situation. The best we're going to get is a state of diminished pain. Face it, we're doomed.

But are we?

What Is Your Baseline Emotional Tone?

In order to experience good feelings and enhanced mental powers, we must understand what it takes to boost certain neurotransmitters while lowering others. Some people know this intuitively and act on that knowledge with great effectiveness. When they begin to feel low, they know just the kinds of activities that put them back in balance and promote positive feelings. But these people are a tiny minority. Most of us have the kinds of coping skills that Thelma has, and consequently we settle for reducing pain rather than increasing positive emotions.

The first step in the process of boosting intellectual performance and promoting feelings of joy, inner peace, and well-being is to understand your own underlying emotional tone. You have a familiar set of feelings that you regard as normal and even optimal under routine, everyday circumstances. By "optimal," I mean that this feeling state is your preferred condition, just as Thelma preferred being at least mildly depressed. This preference is actually created in your brain by precise amounts of dopamine, norepinephrine, acetylcholine, GABA, and serotonin. I call this specific arrangement of neurochemicals that creates your general underlying feelings your *baseline neurotransmitter level,* or simply the *baseline.*

All of us seek to maintain our baseline. We engage in behaviors that maintain the chemical balance in our brains that creates feelings that are familiar and normal—normal, that is, for us. The underlying emotional tone that is normal for you probably will be quite abnormal for your neighbor. Remarkably, we maintain our baseline no matter how it actually feels. One or another of your neurotransmitters may be relatively excessive or deficient, causing any number of psychological conditions, including sluggish mental functioning, low-level depression, or low-level anxiety. Nevertheless, the brain regards this configuration of chemicals as optimal, primarily because *it's what the brain is used to experiencing.*

In general, whenever neurochemical levels rise above the baseline, they create feelings of excitation. When neurochemicals are considerably elevated, they can give rise to anxiety, hysteria, and manic behaviors. Chemical changes that fall below baseline usually result in feelings of depression and fatigue. If you regard low-level depression as normal, you will engage in behaviors that maintain your low-level depression and will try to avoid situations that cause anxiety, nervous tension, and fear. If you regard anxiety as the norm, you will engage in behaviors that maintain a low level of anxiety because you find depression particularly threatening.

Maintaining Your Baseline, for Better or for Worse

Our brains and nervous systems have long been conditioned to accept and identify with certain feeling states produced by our baseline neurochemical array. One of the primary creators of your baseline was the underlying emotional tone of your family of origin, in which an emotional atmosphere was created that established your brain chemistry patterns. Thelma's family, for example, was consistently depressed. With that depression came many related characteristics, such as passivity and lack of will-power. This atmosphere of depression helped to establish Thelma's baseline, which was characterized by low serotonin levels.

Once our baseline is established, we tend to take it for granted. Indeed, we may not recognize it as different from anyone else's; and if we do, we may simply say, "This is what it feels like to be me." We then maintain that condition of being "me" by maintaining our respective baseline brain chemistry.

Whatever your baseline emotional tone may be, you regard those feelings as safe. Foreign feelings—even those that are wonderful, such as emotions that arise out of intimacy, friendship, and love—seem threatening, simply because they suggest possibilities that you cannot predict. Familiar feelings delude us into thinking that we can predict future events. We believe that we know the kinds of events that will come out of such feelings. And knowing the feelings and the events— even when they are violent or horrible—is somehow better than not knowing them. This is partly why people often remain stuck in relationships and behavior patterns that, by all outside appearances, are destructive or painful.

For example, a few years ago, a fourteen-year-old boy named Jim was referred to me by his physician for compulsive behavior, hyperactivity, and stimulant-drug abuse. I soon learned that Jim's father had verbally and physically abused him when he was a child. This caused Jim's baseline neurochemistry—the neurochemical profile that his brain recognized as normal—to be low in serotonin and high in dopamine, the neurotransmitter that creates feelings of alertness, fear, muscle tension, and all the symptoms of the fight or flight. Jim was always on red alert. (If you have encountered abused children or adult children of alcoholics, you will recognize this as a very familiar condition.) Jim regards this state of arousal and anxiety as the norm. Because these feelings were so familiar, they appeared to Jim as safe. As far as Jim was concerned, life was unpredictable and dangerous and he had to stay on the alert, which meant he had to keep his dopamine levels up lest he lose his vigilance and fall prey to an unexpected attack. As a result, Jim engaged in activities that sustained this state of arousal on a daily basis. He was hyperactive and compulsive; he cut up in class and generally acted out. Though very intelligent, Jim couldn't sit still long enough to study anything, and consequently was labeled a poor student. From Jim's perspective, he was doing just what he needed to do to remain safe and normal; but from the perspective of his teachers, he was out of control.

Since Jim's baseline dopamine levels were relatively high, he didn't experience excitement until his dopamine got really elevated. On those occasions when Jim was looking for a thrill, he had to go to great lengths to get his dopamine levels up high enough to experience excitement. He did this by participating in activities that were extremely arousing, dangerous, and sometimes even life-threatening. Indeed, it was this need for extreme arousal that caused Jim to be attracted to stimulant drugs.

Jim's case was further complicated by the fact that in addition to having high dopamine, he had low serotonin. This made treatment somewhat problematical because if we lowered Jim's dopamine levels, he would experience the effect of his low serotonin, which is depression. Jim would do anything to avoid feeling depressed. He avoided this pitfall by being hyperactive, which maintained his high dopamine, kept him in a state of constant arousal, and masked his underlying depression.

Thelma and Jim are entirely different baseline types, both of which are imbalanced and causing behavioral disorders. Thelma's baseline consisted of both low serotonin and low dopamine. She was depressed and lethargic. If we raise Thelma's dopamine, she's going to experience more energy, aggression, and stress; unfortunately, those feelings overwhelm and terrify her. Put Thelma on a roller-coaster ride and her dopamine levels will skyrocket, but she'll hate that experience. On that same roller-coaster, Jim will be hanging halfway out of the car and demanding that somebody speed up the ride. On the other hand, give Thelma a book and a safe, quiet place to sit and she's perfectly content, even blissful. Give Jim a book and have him sit in that same place and he feels like a caged animal, on the brink of a terrifying depression. Only one of these people exhibits what most people consider socially acceptable behavior, though Jim was no more imbalanced than Thelma. His imbalance was just different from Thelma's.

Though we use the word "depression" in Jim's case as well as Thelma's, their respective depressions are very different from one another. When Thelma gets depressed, she becomes vegetative. She withdraws, eats sugar, and sits in front of the television set or reads a book. Thelma's combination of low serotonin and low dopamine makes her both depressed and inactive. When Jim gets depressed, he still has relatively high dopamine, which means that he will be depressed, anxious, and aggressive. Jim's depression leads to violence, especially against himself.

Sigmund Freud pointed out that those who commit suicide are actually turning their aggression inward. This is clearly supported by the brain-chemistry model. If Jim gets sufficiently depressed, he'll feel like driving his car too fast, playing with explosives, or in one way or another tempting fate. If Jim commits suicide, he'll do it in a particularly violent manner, perhaps by blowing his brains out. On the other hand, when Thelma gets really blue, she might consider suicide but she's not likely to do it, simply because she has little aggression, even against herself, and hates violence. If she does get so low that she attempts suicide, she's likely to do it in the least painful, most antiseptic way possible, such as by taking an overdose of sleeping pills.

Treatment of Jim included lowering his dopamine and elevating his serotonin. As his serotonin levels increased, he began to experience feelings of well-being. Jim wasn't entirely comfortable at first with these feelings; they were foreign and he had to learn to trust them. But with time and consistent behavior, Jim began to enjoy feeling good. Gradually, he allowed himself to be more restful, relaxed, and better able to concentrate.

Without treatment, Jim's life was headed for a predictable outcome. If he continued to maintain high dopamine levels at baseline, he probably wouldn't be able to sit still long enough to develop the skills that would give him a job and land him in a career. His need to keep his dopamine levels up made him a perfect candidate for cocaine addiction. In short, Jim was headed for trouble. Yet he could no more be considered a "bad" person than Thelma. His brain chemistry was simply out of balance.

Fortunately, we can change our baseline brain chemistry as we overcome one addiction or automatic behavior or another and regain control of our lives. Unfortunately, most of us do not realize how dependent we are on certain substances, behaviors, and foods. All we know is that these behaviors make us feel good; they give us a reward. Let's take a closer look at how the brain maintains its baseline.

Endorphins: How the Brain Rewards You for Certain Behavior

Your brain rewards you for engaging in behaviors that reinforce your baseline. That reward is a sense of well-being, which is communicated in two ways: The first occurs whenever you experience certain compatible and familiar feelings. For Thelma, those feelings were relaxation and satiation; for Jim, they were alertness, aggression, and excitement. The second way is by producing endorphins.

Endorphins are naturally occurring opiates, similar in molecular structure to morphine and heroin, which are produced and released in your brain when you engage in behaviors that the brain enjoys. In effect, the brain produces reward chemicals that give you a kind of opiumlike high every time you do something that the brain recognizes as good.

"We tend to think that heroin addicts live in an artificial land of vapors, while the rest of us experience a 'real world' unclouded by chemicals," writes Judith Hooper and Dick Teresi in their book on the brain, *The Three Pound Universe* (Jeremy P. Tarcher, 1986). "The truth is that there is no such thing as a chemical-free reality. The greatest manufacturer and user of drugs is the human brain. And each of us is subtly altering our brain chemistry—and our reality—all the time."

Thus the long-distance runner, meditator, and morning-coffee drinker have at least one thing in common: They are all getting rewarded for their behavior through the release of endorphins in their brains.

Endorphins, which are part of a larger family of chemicals called neuropeptides, are involved in such a wide array of chemical events inside your nervous system that it's nearly impossible to catalog them all. In general, they reduce and even eliminate pain and promote feelings of well-being. They are released during exercise and are responsible for the well-known "runner's high" experienced by long-distance runners. They are also released during meditation, prayer, or whenever you listen to your favorite music. Studies have shown that even small amounts of alcohol cause the release of endorphins into the bloodstream, and that heavy drinkers may suffer from an inability to produce adequate quantities of endorphins, which may promote their intake of alcohol to artificially stimulate the production of these reward chemicals. Excessively high levels of endorphins have been found in the blood of people suffering from anorexia (which may explain the reward anorexics get from not eating) and in the blood of schizophrenics—in fact, they are sometimes given the endorphin-blocking drug Naloxone to reduce the frequency of hallucinations. Endorphins are also involved in the stimulation of sexual response and sleep. In general, they promote feelings of safety and pleasure. Indeed, many scientists believe that without endorphin release, we couldn't experience any kind of pleasurable sensation at all.

Dipping Below the Baseline

As we've seen, familiar feelings and endorphins provide you with a reward every time you reinforce or reestablish your baseline. And as we will see in the next chapter, you get additional rewards for behaviors that heighten your baseline and promote feelings that are in line with your general personality type. When you dip below your baseline, however, you automatically want to engage in certain kinds of behaviors to reestablish your baseline, and often crave a particular food

For people with baselines like Thelma's, a further drop in serotonin levels or an elevation in dopamine triggers the need to eat carbohydrates (whole grains or pasta, for example) or simple sugars (in the form of ice cream, candy, or cake), watch television, or perhaps drink alcohol. For people with baselines like Jim's that maintain high dopamine levels, the drop in dopamine may trigger the craving for coffee or some other caffeinated beverage, red meat or eggs, or the desire to engage in some highly arousing activity, such as mountain climbing, bungee jumping, or sex. Once the brain gets what it wants, it releases endorphins that the person experiences as rewarding and pleasurable.

Rewards Can Become Addictive

Any behavior, food, or substance that provides a reward has the potential to become addictive, especially since these activities and substances are usually engaged in unconsciously or automatically. Once we are addicted to a substance or activity, we must use it or participate in it to continue getting a reward. Or we may graduate to stronger substances or participate in more of the same kinds of activities in order to maintain the rewarding feeling.

People like Thelma are tempted by alcohol because they are essentially comfortable with depression, they withdraw from stress and arousal, and they are sensitive to the rises and falls of their serotonin levels. People like Jim are tempted by caffeine, cocaine, and thrill-seeking, which raise dopamine levels and promote all those familiar feelings for the dopamine-sensitive people.

It isn't just substance abuse that becomes addicting, however. Behaviors such as anorexia nervosa, perfectionism, or workaholism are also addictions, and they arise in the same way—by providing neurochemical rewards. A few years ago, I appeared on the *Maury Povich Show* with six women, all of whom were addicted to perfectionistic behaviors. These women had low serotonin and relatively higher dopamine levels. This combination caused them constant anxiety and promoted the need to control their environments in the only way they could: by constantly cleaning, keeping order, and preventing anything from leaving its prescribed place. Such behavior promoted the feeling of being in control and provided what little measure of relaxation these women could experience. In fact, their behavior drove their serotonin levels upward, which gave them a reward. Soon they became addicted to the reward, which meant that they had to compulsively keep their environments neat and under control. As with other addictions, the compulsivity had to grow to maintain the rewards. Consequently, what started out as a small addiction—say, keeping a certain part of the house perfectly clean and under control—eventually spread to the rest of the house and beyond to virtually every part of their lives. Other compulsions, such as gambling, function in the same way: They reward for elevating a neurotransmitter, in this case dopamine, and—when the gambler wins—flood the brain with endorphins.

People who engage in repeated behaviors, such as excessive neatness, are attempting to restore balance to their neurochemistry. Essentially, they're trying to medicate themselves. Eventually, these behaviors can become addictive.

Changing the Baseline to Adapt to the Environment

Adaptation is usually considered to be good—we adapt to survive, for example. But there are lots of different ways to adapt to a situation. Indeed, if you place ten people in a highly stressful situation, you may see ten different ways of adapting. Some forms of adaptation may not provide for our long-term health, and may even lead to addiction.

Addictive behavior frequently occurs in stressful situations at work, and for many leads to workaholism. Let's say you get a job that turns out to be very high pressure. You want to excel at the job, even to prove that you can make it in this highly competitive world. Consequently, you work long, hard hours under tremendous tension. These conditions drive your dopamine levels upward, keeping you in a state of arousal and fear—in this case, fear of failure. Over time, however, you get used to these kinds of conditions and even learn to thrive on them.

Your baseline is changing. You are adjusting to higher dopamine levels, which now become the norm. Since this is the expected behavior for the job environment, you are rewarded by colleagues for behaving according to the prevailing standards. You also turn in reports or complete tasks that gain the appreciation of your peers and superiors, which results in further biochemical rewards. The entire environment now has conspired to change your brain chemistry and behavior. You are now a workaholic. Relaxation and feelings of well-being and receptivity are diminished in value in favor of alertness, aggression, high tension, and rapid productivity.

The brain chemistry that works in one environment may not work in another. When you go home to your family, you cannot simply switch gears and be a loving, supportive, and open spouse or parent. Your baseline is addicted to dopamine and norepinephrine. You will need increasingly higher levels of stimuli in order to maintain and exceed the current dopamine levels.

Typically, corporate America couches such addiction in words like "the need for increasing challenges," or "moving up the corporate ladder," or "gaining greater responsibility." All of these phrases actually translate into conditions that will increase dopamine levels and ensure that the addiction remains in place. Unless you make changes in lifestyle that ultimately affect the baseline neurochemistry, you will likely suffer some kind of family or health crisis, because the addiction causes one side of your life to be neglected.

This phenomenon is not limited to the workplace. It is particularly in evidence in our media, where television, films, and video games must provide increasingly powerful images to have the same impact on brain chemistry, and thus continue to draw customers. Cinematic special effects, violence, and sex must be ever more graphic, arousing, exciting, or disturbing in order to achieve new levels of excitement and arousal. Eventually, the brain adapts to the higher blood levels of certain neurotransmitters, creating a new baseline. In effect, the bar has been raised, meaning that new films must provide even more hair-raising stunts or even more shocking scenes to create the same levels of excitement that previous films were able to achieve with tamer images. As the images become more stimulating, brain chemistry adapts even further, until only participation in certain kinds of behaviors can create the same experience of arousal. Or, to put it another way, only more powerful experiences can create the feeling of being alive.

Moods, Habits, and the Deeper You

All of this can make us sound like biochemical soup, at the mercy of prevailing conditions at our jobs and within our culture. Fortunately, that is not the case. In fact, we suffer more because this is not the case.

If we could make robots of ourselves, we would have long ago. Instead, our brain chemical imbalances cause us considerable suffering. The brain chemical imbalances that give rise to the workaholic, the compulsive gambler, the chronically depressed, and the thrill seeker cause us considerable hardship and heartache. If we were mere extensions of our brain chemistry—if there wasn't something deeper within us—we would indeed be automatons, having no other inner world but that which our neurochemical imbalances dictate.

This brings me to a crucial point about the relationship between brain chemistry and the mind: The deep part of your being that you know to be your true self, the person you experience when you say "I," *is deeper and more fundamental to your identity than your mood!* Moods, no matter how powerful they may be at affecting the quality of your life, actually ride on the surface of your inner self. They may affect your inner being. They may make you feel this way or that, but they are essentially emotional weather. You get sunny days and you get rainy days, but the "you" who experiences the sun and the rain is separate, deeper, and more central to your life than the weather.

When Thelma adopted her program and began to experience relief from her depression and fatigue, she still recognized herself as Thelma. The only difference was that she felt good. She felt like Thelma standing in the sun, as opposed to Thelma standing in the rain. It just felt better to spend more time in the sun than she had in the past.

Most of us, unfortunately, do not make this distinction. The line between mood and identity gets so blurred that we begin to identify too closely with how we feel rather than with who we are. We make judgments about ourselves, such as, "I am a depressed person" or "I am an anxious person." This identification with a negative mood state can become a serious problem because it makes us afraid to change. We want to be happy, but we secretly worry that the changes we'd have to make may cost us our identity.

Don't worry. The inner you is still you, no matter whether you're feeling up or down. When you're feeling good, you experience *you* feeling good. When you're feeling down, you experience *you* in a low mood. The *you* beneath the mood is the experiencer, the true self, which can grow without losing your sense of self. However, the wave line that describes your emotions changes a great deal, like the weather.

I prefer to feel good, so—as much as I can—I do the things in my life that make me feel good. That way, I feel good a lot more than I feel bad. You can do the same—without ever losing the deeper connection with who you are.

Change begins with the understanding that *your moods are not you*. As you go on to recognize the consistent underlying emotional weather patterns that you experience every day, you can begin to work on them consistently to change your baseline.

In the next chapter, you'll find out how to determine whether your emotional tone tends toward a Satiation personality or an Arousal personality, the two general behavioral categories into which everyone fits. Once you have identified your personality type, you can begin to take steps that lead to balance.

3

Arousal or Satiation?

Finding Your Basic Personality Type

Most of us prefer to be either aroused or relaxed as a general condition, depending on our baseline neurochemistry—the feelings we recognize as normal. Most of us are one of two types—either an Arousal type or a Satiation type. Knowing which of the two you are is the key to adopting an effective program for feeling great and reaching your potential.

Generally, *Satiation personalities* prefer to feel sated and relaxed. They seek out foods, activities, and situations that increase brain levels of serotonin, which provides a sense of safety, relaxation, and satiation. They will also behave in ways that inhibit the excitation neurotransmitters dopamine and norepinephrine. Conversely, *Arousal personalities* prefer to be excited, aroused, and in a heightened state of alertness. They will adopt behaviors that increase brain levels of dopamine and norepinephrine while decreasing serotonin, in order to experience a more consistent state of arousal.

Not only do we prefer to feel *either* arousal or satiation, but any prolonged experience of the non-preferred condition will create anxiety or depression. Thus for Satiation types, any prolonged state of arousal can be disturbing and even threatening. For Arousal types, however, prolonged states of calm or satiation create anxiety and depression.

The Arousal and Satiation types are nicely illustrated by Jim and Thelma, who represent extremes on the spectrum. Jim is a classic Arousal type personality. Thelma is a classic Satiation type personality. Our own tendencies may not be as well defined as Thelma's and Jim's, but most of us are more of one than the other.

Most of us experience satiation and arousal conditions to varying degrees during any particular day. Indeed, we choose to be more aroused in the morning in preparation for the work day ahead. This causes many of us to consume caffeinated beverages and protein-rich foods for breakfast, both of which will promote brain levels of dopamine and norepinephrine. These substances will help us feel alert, excited, and aroused to meet the demands of the day ahead. At the end of the day, however, we prefer foods and activities that do the opposite: promote satiation, relaxation, and sleep. What we're really trying to do is increase brain levels of serotonin. The foods that will do that best are those rich in carbohydrates, especially sweets, and alcohol. Activities that will promote serotonin production include watching television, reading, talking, soft music, and taking an evening stroll.

Still, there are degrees of preference for arousal and satiation, and it is impossible to avoid having some degree of both. Anyone who works for a living and must meet a production schedule will be aroused to some degree, and everyone must rest. Most of us enjoy periods of arousal during the average day, or for part of a given work cycle. We also actively pursue quiet, reflective periods, especially when facing a major decision. At face value, these may appear to be contradictions in our temperament; but as you will see, such contradictions actually prove the rule. In any case, the key questions in determining where you fall on the biochemical spectrum are these:

- What activities do you prefer to engage in when you are free to decide how you're going to use your time, such as at night or on weekends?

- How do you prefer to feel during those times — aroused and excited, or satiated and relaxed?

- What do you do for relaxation and to boost your self-esteem? Do you find ways to stimulate yourself, or do you withdraw from stimulation?

The questionnaire at the end of the chapter will help you determine your baseline neurochemistry and whether you are an Arousal or Satiation type personality. But first let's look at a profile of the two types.

The Satiation Type Personality

People whose brain chemistry selects for satiation will seek out foods and activities that boost serotonin and GABA levels. These neurotransmitters provide relaxation, feelings of well-being, and very often improved concentration and mental clarity. Behaviors that raise serotonin and GABA support the Satiation personality's baseline neurochemistry, thus restoring feelings of security and normalcy. Therefore foods and activities that support this baseline and trigger a reward become directly related to a feeling of comfort. These behaviors promote positive self-esteem, even though they may appear negative to someone with an Arousal type personality.

Satiation people generally fall into the "Type B" personality group, people who emphasize relationships over ambition or goals (the exact opposite of the "Type A" personality). Satiation types like lengthy, intimate, and intellectual conversations, as opposed to emotional discussions full of passion and conflict. They can take limited risks with their emotions, but do not enjoy physical danger, stress, or insecurity of any kind. They are prone to perfectionism and controlling behaviors. They attempt to control their environments—often in subtle and passive ways—in an effort to gain some degree of comfort.

Satiation types are good team players who want to blend with others and achieve group goals, but they do not enjoy working in large groups. They prefer intimacy over group dynamics. Whenever groups become larger than four or five, Satiation types feel insecure and begin to withdraw. Large groups are too stimulating, too competitive, too unpredictable, and too demanding on an interpersonal level for the Satiation type.

Generally, Satiation types are attracted to carbohydrate-rich foods, especially foods rich in simple sugars, which increase brain levels of serotonin. They enjoy beer and wine and use both to relax. They are especially drawn to alcohol after a stressful day on the job or when dealing with emotional conflict. Consequently, they can easily be drawn into alcoholism because of alcohol's powerful ability to increase serotonin levels. Some drink coffee to fortify themselves for the work day. The caffeine and the resulting dopamine rush give them that energetic and emotional push they need to confront work and activities that they would not otherwise enjoy or look forward to. Although this helps them temporarily, many feel anxious later in the day.

Many Satiation types are connoisseurs of fine food and wine. The whole enterprise of shopping for high-quality foods, preparing them in a festive setting, anticipating their pleasures, and enjoying the foods deeply is all geared toward achieving deeper and more satisfying satiation.

People in the Satiation group engage in activities that promote relaxation, such as walking, relaxing at home, and listening to music. They prefer folk music, soft rock, or more meditative classical music, such as Chopin or Bach. Many people with Satiation personalities greatly enjoy reading, though younger Satiation types often gravitate to movies, television, and video games. Satiation types like movies of all types, but they are often drawn to intellectually oriented films. The vast majority of Satiation types use television as an anesthetic, and consequently watch more television than Arousal types, most of whom don't have time for TV.

They exercise by walking (especially in nature), swimming, cross-country skiing, and bicycle riding (on flat surfaces). As a general rule, they do not like competitive sports or highly competitive situations. Satiation types enjoy sports that they play against themselves. Whether it's golf, tennis, skating, or skiing, however, Satiation types usually play the "inner game," emphasizing skill development, emotional equilibrium, and the subtle grace and harmony of movement over the struggle to defeat an opponent.

People who have a Satiation reward center find a small amount of boredom and even depression much more comfortable than a small amount of anxiety or change. They regard a workday that's been full of arousing activities as exhausting and difficult. Naturally, they will often find themselves in conflict with people who need constant stimulation, new challenges, and excitement.

Satiation types are drawn to quiet and meditative religious practices and cannot understand why anyone would enjoy, say, a lot of loud singing in church, emotional homilies, and fire and brimstone imagery. The introversion of Satiation types leads to the more introverted religions.

Satiation people also like emotionally based religious or spiritual belief-systems. They are drawn to such truths as unconditional love, forgiveness, and reconciliation with God. But unlike Arousal personalities, Satiation types take a quieter, more introverted approach to such philosophical beliefs. They hold these truths close to their hearts and turn to them for emotional solace.

Too much stress, excitement, and arousal quickly become destabilizing and threatening to Satiation types. Consequently, they avoid such situations or quickly find ways of escaping them.

The danger facing Satiation types is that they can easily overindulge in foods, alcohol, and activities that support satiation. In other words, they may fail to achieve balance. This is the key to their emotional and psychological health and their success in whatever they do. They must achieve some degree of balance between satiation and arousal.

Satiation types who become too introverted can easily become reclusive, partly because they may come to fear those situations that promote a rise in dopamine and norepinephrine levels. Their retreat into satiation threatens to weaken their self-confidence and lead them to believe that they are too weak to handle the stress and strain of conflict. That lack of confidence stems from an intuitive awareness that their own brain levels of dopamine and norepinephrine are low. These neurotransmitters provide strength, alertness, vitality, and the willingness to fight for what one believes to be right. Without such an inherent sense of personal power, Satiation types can easily become depressed and overwhelmed by life, and overwhelmed and victimized by their circumstances.

Satiation types are also prone to various types of compulsions and addictions. Excessive indulgence in satiation-inducing foods (such as sugar), drinks (such as alcohol), activities (such as television watching), and drugs (such as marijuana, sleeping pills, or tranquilizers) lead eventually to dependencies and addiction. The Satiation type can indulge in compulsive behaviors, such as overeating, perfectionism, and various kinds of withdrawal from society.

Satiation types want to be supported and nourished by someone or something that is stronger than they are. They are looking for protection, comfort zones, safety, and a sense of well-being. When they cannot find these feelings in themselves, they will look for them in others. This can lead to dependency on a strong ideology or strong leader. Satiation types with particularly low serotonin can fall under the spell of a charismatic leader, or fringe religious or political group.

For these reasons, it's important for Satiation types to have rewarding work, engage in regular exercise, and recognize how essential it is to participate fully in all the struggles of daily life. Such struggles maintain balance and strength, and support the Satiation person's sense of self-esteem. The knowledge that they can enter conflict and emerge victorious is an essential balance against their natural tendency toward comfort, relaxation, and withdrawal. Balance is the key to the health and well-being of the Satiation type.

Personality Traits

- Generally introverted. Prefers close friendships that are maintained over long periods, as opposed to new and exciting associations.
- Promotes production of inhibitory neurotransmitters, serotonin and GABA.
- Has difficulty letting go of old relationships, old job.
- Is very attached to daily routine.
- Relationship oriented.
- Family centered.
- Moderate to low ambition.
- Avoids conflict. Will repress anger; avoids expressing feelings that may cause antagonism.

Types of Work Preferred

- Office work, preferably done alone or in small groups.
- Work with low physical demands.
- Jobs that do not involve high stress (unless stress is internally created as a drive for success).
- Jobs with regular working hours, with weekends, holidays, and birthday off (unless internal drives cause workaholism).
- Computer technician.
- Librarian.
- Homemaker.
- Teacher, preferably of kindergarten and lower grades, or college (most college professors are Satiation types).

- Research scientist.
- Pediatrician, family doctor, internist, or general practitioner (as opposed to emergency room physician or surgeon).
- Consultant.

Foods Preferred

- Sugar.
- Sweet, carbohydrate-rich foods, such as bakery items, Danish, croissants, muffins, cakes, donuts.
- Candy (soft).
- Chocolate.
- Peanut butter and other nut butters.
- Fruit.
- Sweet dairy foods, such as ice cream, milkshakes, frozen yogurt.
- Soft dairy foods, such as milk and soft cheeses like Brie and Camembert.
- Pasta.
- Soft grains, such as boiled rice, wheat, and barley.
- Beer.
- Wine.
- Hard liquors.
- Typical breakfast choices: tea or coffee with sweet roll, or white roll with butter.
- Typical lunch choices: soft drink, salad, turkey sandwich, chicken salad sandwich, sweet dessert.
- Typical dinner choices: macaroni and cheese, pasta primavera, chicken and fish, rice and sautéed vegetables.

Types of Exercise Preferred

- Walking.
- Stretching.

- Swimming.
- Low-impact aerobics.
- Long-distance running.

Types of Entertainment Preferred

- Films: love stories, romantic dramas, comedies, foreign films, and light feel-good movies.
- Dinners out in intimate settings.
- Long talks.
- Museums.
- The symphony.
- The theater: intellectual dramas and feel-good musicals.
- Music preferences: Soft (folk, light rock, meditative classical music, easy listening).

Vacations and Vacation Activities Preferred

- Low activity, high relaxation, such as lying on a beach.
- Time with family at a private beach or in country setting where there is little to do, few demands, and few people to interfere with relaxation.
- Places where time slows down.

Recreational or Prescription Drugs Preferred

- Marijuana.
- Barbiturates.
- Antidepressants, such as Prozac.
- Anti-anxiety, such as Valium, Xanax, others.
- Sleeping pills (over-the-counter or prescription).

Best Forms for Achieving Insight

- One-on-one counseling.
- Counseling within small groups of two or three.

- Talking-based, rather than activity-based.
- Religion and spiritual practices: low arousal, highly meditative, relaxing, internal.
- Self-help books and tapes.

The Arousal Type Personality

People whose neurochemistries select for Arousal seek out foods and activities that boost the gas-pedal neurotransmitters, dopamine and norepinephrine. These neurotransmitters increase energy and aggression; boost muscle coordination, raise heart rate, increase metabolism, and quicken respiration; heighten awareness and alertness; at higher levels, they trigger the familiar fight-or-flight response. At the extreme, they can lead to paranoia, chronic anxiety, and violence.

Arousal types experience peace of mind, feelings of normalcy, and neurochemical rewards when they are busy, active, and deeply involved in the hustle and bustle of daily life. They love excitement, change, new horizons, and new people to meet. Essentially, they are always looking for stimulation. Arousal personalities are often information and news junkies; many are acutely aware of current trends, fashion, and the latest developments in their fields. They love to work, play, and party. Since they are continually promoting dopamine and norepinephrine release, they tend to be highly energetic. Arousal types enjoy travel and learning about new places and subjects. They are risk-takers. They enjoy carnival rides, fast driving, violent movies, gambling, and sexual conquest. They often lack trust for those around them and consequently do not easily make deep connections with people. They tend to have many acquaintances but little intimacy.

Arousing and exciting activities are often directly tied to the Arousal personality's self-esteem, so that by engaging in an adventure or accomplishing a goal or engaging in some kind of exciting sport, Arousal types feel better about themselves.

Arousal people are often classified as "Type A," but as Jim's example demonstrates, they form a much larger group than is typically defined by Type A. That subset of Arousal people who conform to the Type A description are indeed ambitious, goal oriented, and sometimes workaholics. They are often highly competitive, are driven to succeed, and enjoy taking risks. Arousal types are attracted to jobs that provide stimulation and even conflict. They enjoy having ten things to do at once, and feel trapped and stifled if they don't have such a continual stream of new and exciting projects. Success is of inordinate importance to the self-esteem of Arousal personalities. They enjoy group dynamics and often rise to be leaders within a company. Thus many dynamic and creative leaders are Arousal types.

However, there is another subset of Arousal types who have not been able to channel their energy in socially acceptable patterns. Their need for excitement, thrilling adventures, and risk-taking lead them into dangerous enterprises and eventually to ventures outside the law. Drug dealers—especially cocaine dealers—are uniformly Arousal types who need exceedingly high levels of dopamine to maintain their baselines and feel normal. This pattern occurs because such people established a tolerance to high levels of dopamine and norepinephrine early in life. Consequently, they needed greater degrees of stimulation to feel safe, normal, and rewarded. Many Arousal types, especially those who fall into criminal behaviors, have baselines of high dopamine and low serotonin. This combination makes them aggressive and alert on one hand, but secretly depressed and withdrawn on the other. Their intuitive awareness of their own depression causes them to engage in behaviors and eat foods that continually raise dopamine levels, in part because of their fear of falling into depression and withdrawal. Eventually, tolerance is established even to these high levels, until only the riskiest endeavors provide feelings of excitement, well-being, and self-esteem.

All types of Arousal people are attracted to high-protein foods, which boost dopamine and norepinephrine levels. They must be careful to avoid becoming junk food junkies. They are especially attracted to hamburgers, cheeseburgers, steak sandwiches, red meats, and other unhealthy high-protein foods. These foods give rise to heart disease, cancer, adult-onset diabetes, and other degenerative diseases. Because they boost dopamine and norepinephrine levels, their overconsumption can lead to imbalances in brain chemistry and distortions in perception and outlook.

Arousal types gravitate to recreational activities that tend to be physically demanding, competitive, and adventuresome. They play to win. They particularly enjoy basketball, racquetball, tennis (they couldn't care less about the inner game), mountain climbing, whitewater rafting, skiing (especially downhill), and bicycle riding (also on hills). Arousal types identify with demanding and competitive activities. Pitting oneself against another competitor is highly arousing, meaning that it pumps the body full of dopamine and norepinephrine.

As for entertainment, Arousal types like exciting classical music, such as Beethoven and Tchaikovsky, New Orleans jazz, rock music, heavy metal, and punk. They enjoy vacations on the go, travel to exotic locations with lots of activity.

Arousal types have trouble relating effectively to people who enjoy satiation activities, such as calm music, lengthy and intimate conversations, and relaxation. Arousal types are quick to get "antsy," and often don't know how to relax without some exciting activity. They avoid situations that encourage relaxation. In fact, they are afraid of being depressed, alone, or having nothing to do. The alternative is to keep themselves stimulated.

In general, Arousal types tolerate anxiety better than they do boredom or depression. Such tolerance for anxiety allows them to push their own limits, which often leads to chronic stress and acute anxiety.

They are attracted to religions and churches that are also arousing, emotional, and exciting. They love singing and exciting sermons that deal with conflict and contemporary issues. They enjoy the social component of religion, shaking hands during the ceremony, and meetings before and after services. Some Arousal types are drawn to the Pentecostal faith, where people worship with a lot of emotion. Arousal types will take both an emotional and an intellectual approach to religion, but they want to see their faith in action. They like going out into their community and spreading the word to others. Some become missionaries.

Like their Satiation counterparts, Arousal types are prone to their own types of addictions, most notably to alcohol, caffeine, cocaine, sex, violence, work, and compulsive risk-taking, such as gambling. Arousal types are often attracted to alcohol (especially hard liquors) to help them balance their aggression, alertness, and high anxiety levels.

When Arousal types become overly aggressive, they seek to control their environments and those around them in overt and destructive ways. They may promote conflict, even when they don't realize they are doing it. These feelings may stem from a deep lack of trust, insecurity, and even paranoia. Remember that baselines with high dopamine often develop in children who have been frightened or abused at home, or whose parents are workaholics. They respond to these dangerous conditions by attempting to maintain alertness and aggressiveness. However, such high dopamine levels maintain that fight-or-flight mentality even after they leave their home. Often, such perceptions of danger and mistrust are projected on otherwise benign situations, causing unnecessary conflict and even violence.

Personality Traits

- Goal oriented and highly ambitious.
- Generally extroverted. Prefer having many friends, new acquaintances, and new and exciting social situations in which they can meet new people.
- Promote production of excitatory neurotransmitters, dopamine and norepinephrine.
- Have little difficulty letting go of old relationships and getting on with life.

- Enjoy changes in routine and often promote change.
- Difficulty with intimacy and close relationships.
- Difficulty looking inside themselves for the answers.
- Prefer to change their environment rather than changing themselves.
- Tend to emphasize career over family, though this may be unconscious and they may deny this strongly.
- Find conflict stimulating, exciting, and arousing, and may seek it out when they feel justified or when dopamine and norepinephrine are low and need boosting.
- Will experience anger, especially if dopamine levels are low.
- Seek out challenge or stressful situations, crisis, and difficult challenges, though may do so unconsciously.
- Place self-esteem in the achievement of goals and ambitions, which raises the stakes of any undertaking to disproportionately high levels. Thus goals and ambitions often eclipse other priorities in life.

Types of Work Preferred

- Outdoors.
- Jobs requiring physical activity and much change.
- High-stress positions, even those that are relatively low on the ladder.
- Work long hours, weekends, and holidays and are prone to workaholism.
- Police officer.
- Rescue worker.
- Politician.
- Journalist.
- Scientist with bent for public speaking, or highly political positions.

- Social activist.
- Emergency room doctor, surgeon.

Foods Preferred

- Protein-rich foods, such as red meat, hard cheeses, eggs, poultry.
- Coffee.
- Caffeinated soft drinks, such as colas.
- Spicy foods, especially hot spices.
- Exotic foods.
- Typical breakfast: eggs Benedict; eggs and bacon or sausage; steak and eggs; coffee.
- Typical lunch: hamburgers; cheeseburgers; hot dogs; roast beef sandwich; French fries; caffeinated soft drinks.
- Typical dinner: steak, potatoes, glazed vegetables, alcohol, coffee.

Types of Exercise Preferred

- Vigorous exercise.
- Running.
- Highly arousing, aerobic, and high-risk sports: skiing, water skiing, basketball, tennis, racquetball, skateboard riding, bicycling, ice hockey, hang gliding.
- Aerobics to music.

Types of Entertainment Preferred

- Dancing.
- Improvisational theater.
- Parties.
- Karaoke.
- Rock concerts.

- Sporting events, especially football and basketball games, ice hockey, and boxing matches.

Vacations and Vacation Activities Preferred

- Vacations in big cities (especially New York, New Orleans, and San Francisco).
- Big family reunions.
- Group tours to exotic locations around the world.
- African safari.
- Hunting.

Recreational and Prescription Drugs Preferred

- Cocaine.
- Amphetamines (such as methedrine).
- Hard liquor.

When Contradictions Actually Support the Rule

Almost no one is wholly Satiation or wholly Arousal. Most of us are a bit of both. We all search for balance in our lives, and one of the curious effects of balance is that it allows us to do more of what we like to do. Rest permits us to work or play harder. Hard work makes relaxation more rewarding. Balance is often linked to self-esteem. Many people—no matter what type they are—feel that they must earn their relaxation. Too much rest without the work makes us feel unworthy of our leisure.

This same principle applies to the apparent contradictions in behavior that so often turn up in both the Satiation and Arousal types. The consumption of coffee by Satiation types is a good example, as I explained above in the Satiation profile. The consumption of steak and eggs by Satiation types is another example: these foods boost dopamine levels to provide strength and vitality against the concern—

even the fear—of being overwhelmed by aggressive people or demanding events.

On the other hand, Arousal people are often attracted to alcohol, including hard liquors. Yet alcohol provides satiation (alcohol is a highly refined carbohydrate), which would seem to contradict the Arousal personality's needs. On the surface, that's true; but small amounts of alcohol actually balance the extremes of arousal and allow the person to go on enjoying arousing activities. People who enjoy gambling, a highly arousing activity, often drink alcohol. The reason is that alcohol dampens the arousing effects of gambling, which means that the person can engage in more gambling. Without the alcohol, the gambling would push the Arousal personality to the limit, and thus end the gambling or cause some type of physical or mental breakdown.

Opposites do not always contradict. On the contrary, they may be used to reinforce the patterns you really enjoy. So look for those areas where you use satiation or arousal to allow you to enjoy more of what you truly like—either more satiation, or greater arousal.

Opposites Attract

Ironically, Satiation personalities are usually drawn to and eventually marry Arousal types, and vice versa. Two Satiation types often bore one another to tears; there's no one insisting that the two stop talking and get out of the house and go dancing. On the other hand, two Arousal types are equally ill-matched because neither has time for the other; both are usually caught up in their careers or other endeavors and there's no one insisting on deep conversation, intimacy, and a sense of connectedness with one another. Also, Arousal types find it especially difficult to stay at home and care for the children. They're too drawn to the excitement and conflicts of the outside world.

If a Satiation type marries an Arousal type, mutual understanding and communication are the keys to their success as a couple. If one partner insists that the other be like him, or like her, the two people can easily fall into intense conflict and eventually divorce.

Which Personality Type Are You?

In order to help you better understand which general personality type you are, I've provided the following questionnaire. Answer the questions and tally up your answers according to the instructions that follow the questions. This, along with the above information, should help you determine the first level of your neurochemical profile.

Satiation Vs. Arousal Questionnaire

To determine whether you are a Satiation or Arousal type, answer "yes" or "no" to the fourteen questions below. If you're not certain, answer "yes" if the characteristic is generally true of you. Please answer every question.

1. Do you enjoy actively participating and taking an important role in social or job-related activities?
2. Do you like to socialize with groups of more than two or three people?
3. Do you enjoy watching movies or videos or reading books in which violence or horror play a part?
4. Do you get pleasure from drugs (including nicotine and caffeine) or activities that increase your energy level?
5. Do you feel good when you engage in risk-oriented activities (such as driving your car over the speed limit, mountain climbing, hang gliding, or racing)?
6. When you feel stressed, do activities that cause your heart rate to increase relax you and lessen your stress?

7. Do you find it difficult to enjoy being with people, unless there are activities going on or there is a stimulating conversation taking place?

8. Do you like intimate, close communication with a few friends?

9. Do you usually continue to eat even after you are full?

10. Do you eat when you are depressed, anxious, or angry?

11. Do you use alcohol, drugs, meditation, or quiet activities to relax?

12. On the average, do you spend more than 15 hours a week watching television, movies, or reading?

13. When depressed, do you find the need to withdraw for a while to try to increase your energy?

14. Do you spend much of your free time alone?

Scoring: Assign 1 point to each "yes" answer.

1. Add your "yes" answers for questions 1 through 7 and put the total here: _____

2. Add your "yes" answers for 8 through 14 and put the total here:

   _____

If you have more "yes" answers to questions 1 through 7, you are an Arousal personality. If you have more "yes" answers to questions 8 through 14, you are a Satiation personality. If you have equal numbers of "yes" and "no" answers, read the profiles for both and choose the one you feel fits you best.

Now let's take the next step in our journey of self-discovery and examine your automatic behaviors, the activities you do almost as second nature. These will give you a deeper understanding of your behavior and how it affects your brain chemistry.

4

Automatic
Behaviors

*How We Give
Ourselves Rewards*

You can also determine whether you are a Satiation or Arousal personality by understanding your *automatic behaviors*, the activities you turn to unconsciously for rewards—whether you feel depressed or anxious, or you feel like celebrating.

Automatic behaviors provide a *physiological* reward. For the most part, they either raise or lower dopamine, or they boost serotonin. However, though automatic behaviors may provide us with a physiological reward, they can also be *psychologically* distressing.

Let's differentiate between physiological and psychological rewards. As any frequent dieter knows, the only real reward experienced from abstaining from food is psychological. You get on the scale and you've lost a pound or two, and you're happy because you believe your diet is working. You feel better about yourself because your diet is making you lose weight and you believe that you will ultimately reach your goal—significant weight loss and a more attractive appearance. All of this is based on an image you are trying to achieve, an image that is grounded in your psyche. Hence you derive a psychological reward for losing weight. The problem with dieting, however, is that you've been starving yourself for the duration of your diet. Starvation causes physiological distress in the form of hunger pangs and food cravings, some of which may come from the body's need for certain nutrients. Since eating normally gives us a psychological reward, starvation causes psychological distress, as well.

Some automatic behaviors give physiological rewards but psychological distress. Take alcoholism, for example. Alcoholics may experience a physiological reward whenever they drink an alcoholic beverage because alcohol boosts serotonin and thereby increases relaxation and a sense of well-being. But alcoholics may also feel psychological distress because deep inside they know they're indulging their addiction, which may eventually destroy their life. Thus they experience a physiological reward and psychological distress.

Examples of automatic behaviors and their rewards abound. The type of automatic behavior we engage in reveals our personality type. Many Satiation types eat whenever they are depressed in an attempt to boost serotonin and lower dopamine. Consequently, they will eat lots of sweets or carbohydrate-rich foods. Many people eat chocolate whenever they are stressed, as do many women when they are experiencing their menstrual period. Chocolate has several interesting elements that work in harmony to create satiation and well-being: It contains sugar and milk-carbohydrates, both of which boost serotonin; the milk provides a creamy "mouth feel" that is luscious and satiating; and it also contains caffeine, which boosts dopamine and instantly elevates mood by giving an endorphin rush. The endorphins give us a sense of well-being and reward, and combine with the effects of the sugar and serotonin to create a deep sense of well-being. Others drink alcohol (satiating) and still others use drugs like marijuana or heroin or take tranquilizers.

Exercise, which many people rely on to create short-term relaxation, has a dual effect: It burns off dopamine, which is used when exercising muscles, and it elevates serotonin. This causes deep relaxation and satiation. However, the satiation effects of highly arousing exercise are short-lived. Eventually, the dopamine returns, often in elevated quantities, causing a new round of anxiety, which sends the person back to the gym for more exercise. In this way, exercise can become automatic or addictive. Thus intense, highly arousing exercise is usually done by Arousal types.

As the name implies, automatic behaviors are usually unconscious—we do them without really thinking about them. Because automatic behaviors provide physiological rewards, you can easily become dependent on their effects.

Automatic behaviors, such as perfectionism, control, and orderliness, can also become compulsions. These types of behaviors give us a false sense of peace or safety. Disorder or chaos is threatening to most people. However, when we indulge in perfectionism or ritualistic order, we are actually medicating ourselves. Perfectionism, order, and ritual give us the sense that our lives and environments are under control and safe. When we increase feelings of safety, we decrease dopamine and norepinephrine, which in turn decrease anxiety and tension. At the same time, the increase in personal well-being increases serotonin, which then feeds on itself: As serotonin goes up, the resulting positive feelings boost serotonin even further. That's how these behaviors become compulsive or addictive.

What Are Your Automatic Behaviors?

The following questions can help you identify your automatic behaviors. Once you know your automatic behaviors, you can better determine whether you are an Arousal personality or a Satiation type.

These are not questions to score. Just scan the columns, and you'll probably find that you fit into one or the other.

When I've had a bad day and everything seems to be going wrong, I like to:

SATIATION TYPE	AROUSAL TYPE
Eat	Gamble
Drink alcohol	Exercise
Clean the house	Go to an amusement park
Shop till I drop	Dance till I drop
Watch television or play video games	Take physical and dangerous risks

When I've had a great day, when everything seems to be going right, and I feel like celebrating I would like to:

SATIATION TYPE	AROUSAL TYPE
Eat a great meal	Throw a loud, raucous party
Celebrate by drinking with friends	Hit the slot machines
Buy myself something	Dance till I drop
Go off by myself to ponder the future	Take physical and dangerous risks

The following activities are automatic behaviors divided according to Satiation and Arousal personalities. Because these behaviors have such powerful effects on brain chemistry, we can easily become dependent on them, or they can become compulsions. Locate the behaviors that you most engage in, and use that information to get a clearer picture of whether you are a Satiation personality or an Arousal type.

Automatic Behaviors Used by Arousal Personalities

Alcohol usage. Increases serotonin and lowers dopamine. It is used by Arousal personalities to bring down excessively high dopamine and norepinephrine. In this way, alcohol allows the Arousal person to maintain arousal activities. Without the strong serotonin increase and the lowering of dopamine, the Arousal personality would not be able to sustain his or her high-energy, high-excitement lifestyle.

Avoidance. Avoidance is typically associated with Satiation personalities, but there are circumstances in which the Arousal personality will use a specific type of avoidance response to increase dopamine and norepinephrine, and that's doing busy work. Irrelevant expenditure of energy, often in the form of compulsive activity, such as endlessly running errands or filling up one's schedule with trivial tasks, is most often used to burn off dopamine and norepinephrine. It is a nervous or anxious person's way of trying to dampen brain chemistry.

Drug abuse. Arousal personalities who use drugs are attracted to cocaine, which increases dopamine and norepinephrine and thus boosts arousal. Alcohol is often added to compensate for too much dopamine and to try to sleep.

Eating. Most often, eating is used by Satiation personalities to raise serotonin. However, protein foods are used to create arousal and elevate dopamine and norepinephrine levels. People whose diets are mostly composed of protein foods are most often Arousal types.

Exercise. Most often, Arousal personalities use exercise to calm themselves and create relaxation. Vigorous exercise lowers dopamine and raises serotonin, temporarily. However, dopamine typically increases with time so that another round of exercise is needed to bring down dopamine levels again. The net effect of vigorous, highly aerobic exercise—especially competitive sports—is arousing.

Gambling. Arousal personalities use gambling to maintain or raise dopamine and norepinephrine levels.

Hard work. With lots of stress and pressure, hard work is arousing. In general, work increases dopamine and norepinephrine. Workaholics are getting rewards from maintaining high dopamine levels.

Risk-taking. Risk-taking is arousing, and boosts dopamine and norepinephrine.

Sex. Sex initially increases dopamine and norepinephrine upon arousal; orgasm boosts serotonin.

Theft. Theft, which boosts dopamine, is arousing.

Violence. Violence is arousing, and occurs as a result of low serotonin and high dopamine.

Worship. Types of worship that are highly social and may involve singing or a high degree of emotion are arousing.

Automatic Behaviors Used by Satiation Types

Alcohol usage. Alcohol increases serotonin and lowers dopamine and is used by Satiation personalities to maintain or reestablish their baseline.

Approval-seeking. Approval-seeking often occurs as a result of low serotonin. The person needs a sense of safety and security, which occurs when authority figures approve of the person.

Avoidance. Avoidance is used most often by depressed Satiation personalities to prevent increases in dopamine and norepinephrine. People who use avoidance often feel like victims of circumstance, or they feel too weak to affect their situation. Avoidance is an extreme form of passivity. (However, avoidance can be the response used by Arousal personalities with high dopamine who suffer from too much anxiety and fear and can no longer cope with their circumstances.)

Cleaning. Cleaning often becomes compulsive and is typical among people who have a Satiation reward center but suffer from high dopamine. High dopamine levels are uncomfortable for such people. They use cleaning to create order, burn and lower dopamine, and raise serotonin.

Control. Satiation types typically use control to lower dopamine and norepinephrine and raise serotonin.

Drug usage. The Satiation personality uses drugs that produce satiation: alcohol, marijuana, heroin, and barbiturates especially are used to increase serotonin and satiation.

Eating. Most often, Satiation personalities eat to raise serotonin. However, food can be used to boost satiation or arousal. Satiation personalities turn to carbohydrate foods to elevate serotonin levels.

Exercise. Satiation personalities use vigorous aerobic exercise to raise dopamine and norepinephrine to feel more empowered and in control of their lives. However, Satiation types are more frequently attracted to stretching, low-impact aerobics, walking, and other calming exercises that boost serotonin and lower dopamine.

Media fascination. Watching television, reading books, or going to movies boosts serotonin and lowers dopamine.

Perfectionism. Satiation types use perfectionism to lower dopamine and norepinephrine and raise serotonin.

Procrastination. Procrastination stimulates the Satiation reward center, and is used by people who wish to avoid increases in dopamine levels.

Spend or shop. Satiation personalities looking for feelings of well-being and being cared for shop or spend money to raise serotonin levels. Arousal personalities may shop to reward themselves.

Worship. Meditative or contemplative forms of worship boost serotonin and lower dopamine.

What Happens When You Change Your Baseline?

An interesting twist on the Satiation and Arousal dichotomy is that many people are attempting—either consciously or unconsciously—to change themselves from one to the other. Workaholics often start out as Satiation types but work themselves so hard that they eventually develop a high-dopamine and norepinephrine baseline, which they maintain by remaining under intense pressure and taking on projects that are increasingly challenging and filled with pressure. People who are already workaholics may try to develop the other side of their personalities, their music skills or creative sides, which can bring them into their more receptive and more gentle natures. Such a transformation will inevitably lead to higher serotonin levels and a more satiation-oriented reward center.

Whenever we make major changes in personality, we change our neurochemistry. Often we experience withdrawal symptoms when we alter behavior, even when that behavior doesn't include the use of a drug or alcohol. People with compulsive disorders experience withdrawal pressures, just as recovering alcoholics do. These changes occur because brain chemistry is being altered. For those people who are making such changes, it's important to understand what exactly is going on.

Whenever we change our fundamental behavior patterns, there is a transition period that usually brings with it some discomfort. The most common questions people ask when they alter their automatic behavior or give up a compulsion or addiction are these: What is happening in my brain? Why is my need to revert back to my old behavior patterns so strong? Are these strong urges temporary, or will I have to suffer them indefinitely?

My short answer is this: Your baseline brain chemistry is changing, but those urges to revert back to the old behaviors will last only a short time, while you establish a new baseline. The change is affecting the amount of specific neurotransmitters in your brain, and how efficiently your brain handles those chemicals.

The long answer, of course, is somewhat longer. Here it is.

The Role of Adenylate Cyclase

All cells contain energy, and brain cells are no different. Energy is stored in your cells as a molecule called *adenosine triphosphate*, or ATP. In order for your brain to use ATP, and thereby burn energy, it needs the presence of an enzyme called *adenylate cyclase*. ATP exists in the brain as potential energy until is converted by the enzyme adenylate cyclase, which turns the ATP into kinetic energy. So the more active the adenylate cyclase is in a neuron, the more energy is available to that cell.

Your short-term influence over adenylate cyclase is small. The reason is this: the brain's energy levels tend to adjust themselves to maintain the chemical environment that your brain recognizes as normal or baseline.

Energy is used in neurons to convert the chemical neurotransmitter to an electrical charge. That charge fires along the axon of the cell, causing a response to be produced at the end of the axon. The adenylate cyclase determines how much of the chemical neurotransmitter will be converted to an electrical charge, and how strong that charge will be. Your behavior can cause the production of high levels of a certain neurotransmitter, but your brain will regulate how much of that neurotransmitter you utilize by converting only a small portion of it to electrical current. Adenylate cyclase is the regulator that determines how much of the neurotransmitter will be converted. For example, let's say you suddenly produce a lot of dopamine. Your adenylate cyclase will regulate how much of that dopamine will be converted to a charge, and thus how much dopamine you will experience. So adenylate cyclase regulates the amount of neurotransmitter to be converted according to what your brain regards as normal.

Let me give you a practical example of how adenylate cyclase works. Let's say that Joanna has high norepinephrine and dopamine levels and suffers from anxiety. In order to cope with that anxiety, she begins to indulge in compulsive behaviors. She becomes perfectionistic about her home. Everything must be in its proper place. She also controls her schedule, her appointments, and her relationships in an effort to keep conflict at a minimum. All of this compulsive behavior causes her dopamine levels to fall, which feels good. Now she feels safer and more secure, which reinforces her compulsivity. To her mind, compulsion is working.

Now a strange thing happens. Joanna's neurons recognize that dopamine and norepinephrine levels have fallen below normal baseline, so the cells adjust to make more efficient use of the existing dopamine and norepinephrine. They do this by raising adenylate cyclase efficiency, so that there is more energy in the cell to convert the existing dopamine and norepinephrine to electrical charges. Even though dopamine and norepinephrine levels have fallen, the increase in adenylate cyclase activity actually makes these diminished quantities just as potent because they are utilized more efficiently. Now Joanna's brain chemistry has been restored to what her brain considered normal before the mitigating effects of the compulsive behavior.

Suddenly, her compulsive behavior is not working as well as it used to. She experiences this new condition as an increase in anxiety, which only encourages her to be even more compulsive. Her increase in compulsive behavior does, in fact, lower her dopamine and norepinephrine levels even further; but once again, adenylate cyclase adjusts upward to restore the normal baseline. This, of course, only encourages Joanna to become more compulsive. But adenylate cyclase adjusts again. And that is precisely how compulsive behavior leads to even more compulsivity. Just as with all other forms of addiction, the person needs more of the addictive substance — or behavior — to get the same reward.

Now let's say Joanna attempts to stop being so compulsively neat and controlling. The minute she stops the behavior, dopamine and norepinephrine shoot right back up to their previous normal levels. However, the adenylate cyclase has not had time to adjust, so it remains highly efficient. That means that there is an increase in gas-pedal neurotransmitters, along with an increase in the efficiency with which they are utilized. The net effect is that Joanna experiences extremely high levels of anxiety, fear, insecurity, and paranoia. Her valiant attempt to stop her compulsion has had the same effect as throwing gasoline on a fire. She is overwhelmed by the dramatic increase in dopamine and norepinephrine.

In fact, this is a temporary increase in discomfort, because the adenylate cyclase will eventually adjust downward to restore normal baseline. In other words, it will stop utilizing so much of the dopamine and norepinephrine and thus reduce her anxiety and insecurity. However, since Joanna doesn't realize what is taking place, she feels overwhelmed by her inner turmoil. Her natural reaction is to return to her compulsive disorder, simply because it was the only thing that gave her some relief from her inner pain.

Dealing with Change

It is possible to deal effectively with the ups and downs of conscious change. Here's what you have to do:

First, you'll need to bring down your norepinephrine and dopamine levels gradually, while at the same time increasing serotonin and GABA. This will lower anxiety while increasing feelings of well-being and safety. You can accomplish both of these steps by increasing satiation.

Second, you'll need to maintain the healing behaviors consistently so that a new baseline can be established. The healing effects of time and consistency are an essential part of the healing process. Without such consistent behavior, you will have difficulty establishing a new baseline.

Third, you must understand what is actually taking place within yourself. Without such knowledge, you can easily revert back to the old behavior, because that behavior was the only tool that effectively relieved the terrible stress.

Finally, you will need the support of others for your change in behavior.

Change is never easy, but the brain-chemistry model shows us how to make the desired changes as efficiently and as painlessly as possible. Follow the recommendations provided in this book; try to achieve a balanced brain chemistry by eating foods and practicing behaviors that boost serotonin and moderate dopamine according to your specific personality needs. And stay focused on your goals.

Remember, the brain is the tool of your higher consciousness and your spirit—and not the other way around. In the next chapter, you'll learn how you can maximize your brain's efficiency.

5

Reaching Peak Performance

Quick and Easy
Ways to Maximize
Brain Efficiency

You can approach heightened mental performance in two ways: short-term and long-term. You can boost mental alertness and dexterity almost immediately by altering your brain chemistry temporarily—for example, in order to be alert and efficient at a business meeting. But you can also maintain a lifestyle that supports optimal brain chemistry *all the time*. If you practice the long-term method, which is what I advise, the short-term methods will be much more effective because your brain will be more sensitive and receptive to them.

You can also use these tools to relieve unpleasant moods, as well as anxiety and depression. The short-term tools will help you relieve disagreeable moods; the long-term approach will help you establish a healthy brain chemistry that will allow you to function at your peak. We'll explore these methods at the end of this chapter. First, however, we'll take a look at what controls peak performance.

What Controls Our Neurotransmission Speed?

On several occasions, people have come to me privately and said that they don't feel as mentally sharp any more. "Sharp?" I asked my friend. "What do you mean?"

"My thoughts are slower than they used to be," he told me. "I have to labor to get my ideas to come into focus. My brain feels sluggish, as if it's submerged in molasses. Am I getting stupid, or old or . . . *senile*?" The answers to these questions, respectively, are: no, not necessarily, and no, you're probably not senile.

Actually, this is a very common experience. All of us—no matter how old we are—are aware that from time to time our minds seem to be functioning a little more slowly than we're used to experiencing. Usually, we don't think much about the problem. We chalk it up to the fact that we're working too hard; we're tired—burned out. On the other hand, many people experience chronic mental sluggishness. Some observe that they do not think as rapidly or solve problems as quickly as they used to, or would like to. This is not senility or stupidity, however. It is a matter of the efficiency with which your brain is functioning.

The speed of your thoughts, or what I call *neurotransmission speed*, is determined in part by the same neurotransmitters that govern your moods. Some neurotransmitters excite or speed up neurotransmission, meaning they speed up thinking and problem-solving. These chemicals cause the brain to work faster. Other neurochemicals inhibit or slow down neurotransmission. They make the brain more relaxed.

The wave that describes your high and low neurotransmission speeds varies throughout the day, depending on what you eat, whether or not you exercise, and what you are thinking about. You can speed up your neurotransmission within a few minutes, and you can also calm yourself down just as fast.

The relative abundance or deficiency of certain neurotransmitters is only part of what controls the speed and efficiency of your brain, however. The quantity of oxygen your brain receives at any given moment also determines how efficiently your brain works. The less oxygen your brain gets, the slower and less efficiently it will function. Another factor is the amount of energy your brain cells are able to utilize.

Remarkably, all three of these factors—the types and relative amounts of certain neurotransmitters that dominate your brain chemistry; the quantity of oxygen your brain receives; and the amount of energy utilized by brain cells—are influenced directly by your behavior. It's true that in the broadest terms, these factors are also influenced by your genetic makeup. But your genes determine the outside parameters, the outer limits of your brain's powers. Within those parameters, you have a great deal of latitude over how efficiently—or inefficiently—your brain functions.

To a great degree, you control how efficiently your brain works, though you're probably not aware that you're doing it.

How Fast Are Your Thoughts?

When your brain is functioning optimally you feel mentally alert, relaxed, and blessed with an almost pristine clarity. It's a wonderful feeling. On the other hand, a sluggish brain almost feels like you've been drugged. It feels as if your neural network has been replaced by rusty wiring. But there's more to mental clarity than these metaphors.

Chemically, rapid neurotransmission is made possible by a predominance of the excitatory neurotransmitters, dopamine and norepinephrine, combined with relative low levels of the inhibitors, serotonin and GABA. Norepinephrine and adrenaline (an excitatory hormone) are converted from dopamine. So the higher your dopamine levels, the higher your norepinephrine and adrenaline levels likely will be. When

I talk about rapid neurotransmission levels, however, I'm generally talking about norepinephrine.

We've all experienced how neurotransmitters cause our thoughts to speed up and slow down. Think back to the last time you were excited or afraid. The instant you were aroused, your brain levels of dopamine and norepinephrine increased dramatically, causing—among other things—an increase in neurotransmission speed. Thoughts, options, possibilities fired across your brain like lightning across a darkened sky. Conversely, when you begin to relax and unwind at night, dopamine and norepinephrine levels decrease, while serotonin increases, causing neurotransmission to slow. You're not as sharp, as my friend put it. The mind has slowed down and both mind and body relax.

When Neurotransmission Is Too Fast or Too Slow

There are limits and problems at both ends of the transmission-speed spectrum, however. Excessively fast neurotransmission can cause anxiety and nervous tension. People with excessively fast neurotransmission often lack receptivity and have trouble listening to others. They also tend to be preoccupied with their own ideas, which are firing at a rapid rate. They can be very creative, but they often lack focus and direction. Their ideas often lack unity, as well. Their patience with others decreases. Eventually, these people burn out if they do not make balance with their overabundance of dopamine and norepinephrine.

Excessively slow neurotransmission is associated with mental fatigue, a lack of creativity, and depression. The slower the neurotransmission, the less excitement the person has for his or her ideas—or anyone else's ideas, for that matter. These people often feel like they're in a fog. They feel withdrawn and separated from others. People with really slow neurotransmission can have an enervating effect on others. They don't give much back and can be a drain on a creative process. Both excessively fast and excessively slow neurotransmission can be disturbing.

The Dark Side of Speed

People who are generally balanced in their neurotransmission—meaning that they are able to oscillate between fast neurotransmission and slow, depending on the circumstances—have the clarity to know their own limits. They know when to calm down and concentrate on a particular subject or problem. Most of us, however, have to be trained to recognize that balance is the goal and that too much neurotransmission tends to backfire.

As we saw in the previous chapter, overly ambitious people often have excess dopamine and norepinephrine. Driving oneself to work harder and be more alert in demanding situations can easily push you into workaholism, in part because you can get hooked on the physiological and psychological rewards that flow from high dopamine and norepinephrine, and on high neurotransmission. Many people thrive on pressure and conflict; some believe they can hardly live without it. Consequently, these people are constantly trying to keep up their norepinephrine levels. They get rewards for maintaining high neurotransmission. On the positive side, these people are creative and often full of insight. But they are also like popcorn machines, springing forth new ideas at random. Many people with excessively rapid neurotransmission find it difficult, if not impossible, to slow down and remain focused on any single subject for very long. These are people of action. They thrive on it, which means they are continually pumping gas-pedal neurotransmitters into their brain chemistry.

Unfortunately, too much norepinephrine can rob a person of all the positive aspects that a more balanced or slightly elevated neurotransmission provides. Only you know your limits, but you must respect them if you want to be a healthy and balanced human being.

You may be seduced into believing that one or two more cups of coffee will give you the edge you're looking for; just a little more activity will give you a little boost; just one more project or just a little more pressure and you'll really be cruising. But as Napoleon learned in the snows of Russia, you cannot advance forever. Eventually, unrelenting ambition backfires.

As people's dopamine and norepinephrine levels rise beyond their tolerance, their thoughts and behavior become more scattered and unpredictable. They are less able to focus or concentrate on any single thought or subject for an extended period of time. They will likely have trouble thinking through problems. They become increasingly restless and impulsive; they leap before they look. Why? Because the increase in dopamine and norepinephrine has caused an increase in oxygen levels within the blood, which in turn causes an increase in energy. But that heightened energy is fueled in part by high levels of anxiety. They may also have trouble getting adequate and restful sleep. They are likely to obsess over problems well into the night. Fear and insecurity escalate. So, too, do compulsivity, perfectionism, and workaholism. Eventually, the brain becomes tired. Neurotransmission slows. They cannot think as clearly anymore. At this point, they are usually faced with several possibilities. Either they take a rest and restore balance to their lives, or they keep pushing and suffer from some kind of illness, or start taking drugs. Cocaine is the drug of choice for people who are pushing the neurotransmission envelope to its maximum. Of course, drug addiction merely postpones the inevitable crash that is actually far worse than if they merely had taken some time off and restored balance to life earlier in the process.

Exceedingly rapid neurotransmission is particularly troubling in children, and often causes hyperactivity and attention-deficit disorders. Children with rapid neurotransmission have great difficulty concentrating on any particular idea or subject for more than a few moments. They experience increased muscle activity, insecurity, and excessive restlessness. Their restlessness is fueled in part by a need for some sense of safety—within themselves and their environment—but nothing seems safe, comfortable, or rewarding.

In both adults and children, the answer to the problem of unrelenting and rapid neurotransmission is to slow things down, to become more receptive and open up to a larger view of life.

A good example of someone with rapid neurotransmission is the famous English detective Sherlock Holmes. Holmes, of course, is a genius, a man who sees relationships between events and puts facts together instantaneously. He's quirky, a bit eccentric, and his singular means of turning off his endlessly churning mind is the opium pipe.

Slowing Down the Engine and Focusing the Mind

Slow neurotransmission is the result of low levels of dopamine and norepinephrine, or higher levels of the inhibiting neurotransmitters, serotonin and GABA. Just as rapid neurotransmission is desirable at times, so too is slowing down. When neurotransmission slows, the mind enjoys greater powers of concentration. You are able to settle down and focus on the issue at hand. Slower and more focused neurotransmission is ideal when you're trying to think through a problem, plan a project, or take into account a wide variety of contingencies.

People with slightly slow neurotransmission tend to take a more methodical approach to problem-solving. Ideally, slowness will result in a painstaking approach and considering a wide array of factors in any decision. "He leaves no stone unturned" is usually what is said about a person with slow neurotransmission. Usually, people with slow neurotransmission are not personally aggressive—indeed, they tend to take an objective role in the decision-making process—but like the proverbial tortoise, they will often finish the race with fewer mistakes than their faster counterparts.

People with slower neurotransmission tend to be Satiation types. They are often lovers of music and art. They linger over their pastimes and their loves. They garden, write poetry, and take a gentle approach to life. Consequently, they enjoy gourmet foods, fine wines, and intimate conversation—all of which will slow neurotransmission levels.

The danger they face is overindulgence in foods and activities that promote satiation and slow neurotransmission. If they persist in these behaviors, and avoid balancing their tendency toward satiation, they will become increasingly lethargic, both mentally and physically. They will lack creativity and gradually lose confidence in their mental abilities. Overindulgence in satiation will cause them to suffer low physical energy. They'll lack initiative. They will experience greater passivity and start to believe that they lack the personal power to push projects to completion. Eventually, they will suffer from depression.

Slow neurotransmission speed is not bad of itself. There are many brilliant and gifted people in every walk of life with slow neurotransmission. Slow neurotransmission in a healthy and well-functioning person says more about style and approach to problem-solving than it does about whether or not the person is effective at his or her job. If you compare two equally talented people of opposite types—one with rapid and the other with slow neurotransmission—both will do a job equally well, though they likely will go about their business in very different ways.

An example of someone with moderately slow neurotransmission is the television detective Columbo, played by Peter Falk. He pays little attention to his appearance, he's as slow moving as a snail, and he's utterly self-effacing. He constantly laments his poor memory—he's got to write everything down in his little notebook—and seems late for every appointment he's able to keep track of. Yet he meditates on every fact and every possible clue, and ultimately puts the pieces of the mystery together in creative and resourceful ways. He is Sherlock Holmes's opposite. Yet just as Holmes reveals the positive characteristics of the Arousal personality with rapid neurotransmission, so Columbo demonstrates the brilliance of the Satiation personality with slow neurotransmission.

Ways to Improve Concentration When You're Moving Too Fast

You can slow down neurotransmission and increase your ability to concentrate by eating foods that are rich in carbohydrates. Any snack made up of carbohydrates will create satiation and increase your concentration within minutes of consumption. Some healthful choices include all whole grains, fruit, fruit juice, cookies, rice cakes with jam or apple butter, any type of cereal eaten dry (or use apple juice in place of milk; milk is higher in protein and fat, which will not give you the powers of concentration that you are looking for). Less healthful foods include candy, cakes, and other processed foods.

Two Methods to Help You Achieve Peak Performance

As promised, here are the short-term and long-term ways to achieve greater mental efficacy.

Method 1: Making the Brain Work Faster in Under Thirty Minutes

Peak neurotransmission is associated with arousal, not satiation. When you are peaking, you have the ability to see relationships between ideas and objects quickly and make decisions rapidly. At the same time, you are aware of your mental and physical agility. Your mind is sharp, clear, and nimble. Your body is full of energy, thanks in part to the increased muscle activity and the higher levels of oxygen in your bloodstream—both the result of elevations of dopamine and norepinephrine. All of these are symptoms of arousal.

With these arousal symptoms come a rush of physiological and psychological rewards. Physiologically, those rewards may include the reestablishment of your baseline and a cascade of endorphins. Psychologically, the rewards include feelings of increased self-esteem and the reassurance that you are aggressive, smart, decisive, and alert.

You can raise your norepinephrine levels quickly—usually in less than thirty minutes—to make yourself more alert, keener of mind, and sharper of wit by eating foods that contain protein. Low-fat fish, such as cod, flounder, fluke, halibut, scrod, salmon, and smoked salmon (lox) are ideal. Chicken (preferably range-fed, without steroids

Caffeine Content of Beverages and Foods

Chocolate, 1 ounce (milk chocolate)	6 milligrams
Coffee, percolated	110–170 milligrams/cup *(depending on brewing time)*
Coffee, drip	110–150 milligrams/cup *(depending on brewing time)*
Coffee, instant	120 milligrams/cup
Coffee, decaffeinated	3–4.5 milligrams/cup *(depending on brewing time)*
Coca-Cola	42 milligrams/12 ounces
Dr. Pepper	61 milligrams/12 ounces
Pepsi-Cola	35 milligrams/12 ounces
Diet Pepsi	34 milligrams/12 ounces
Tea, black or green	45–100 milligrams/cup *(depending on brewing time)*

and antibiotics), eggs, and—though less healthful—red meats will all boost tyrosine and dopamine levels. So will tofu and other bean products. Coffee, tea, and other caffeinated beverages will trigger the same response, accelerating neurotransmission speed within minutes.

CAFFEINE: HIGH OCTANE IN A SINGLE CUP

All foods and beverages containing caffeine rapidly increase neurotransmission speed. Studies have shown that coffee, for example, makes people more alert, improves mental acuity and concentration, and dramatically enhances problem-solving abilities. It also elevates mood, boosts confidence, and makes people more optimistic, if only temporarily. Caffeine has an antidepressant effect on mood and may even produce euphoria. These improvements occur across the board, whether people are habitual caffeine consumers, are occasional consumers, or drink it only on rare occasions.

Caffeine also works quickly. As everyone who drinks a morning cup of coffee knows, caffeine gets into the bloodstream and affects brain chemistry within minutes after taking those first few sips. Research has shown that just one or two cups of coffee provide all the brain-boosting you need. The effects of that morning cup of coffee last anywhere from three to five hours, depending upon how rapidly you metabolize the caffeine and eliminate it from your body. Because tea has a much lower caffeine content than coffee (see chart on page 88), it tends to wear off more quickly than coffee.

In any case, those morning cups of coffee or tea will last you into the early afternoon. However, improvements in mood and brain function do not go up endlessly with more caffeine consumption. At a certain point, depending on your tolerance levels, caffeine creates anxiety, loss of concentration, loss of sleep, muscle spasm, and heart arrhythmia. Some studies suggest that coffee may be linked to bladder cancer and fibrocystic breast disease.

The effects of caffeine — both the desired effects and their aftermath — are a perfect example of the pros and cons of using a drug to boost neurotransmission. The first cup of coffee immediately boosts neurotransmission and usually provides the desired endorphin rush. The second cup reinforces it. But the more coffee you drink, the more tense you become, especially after the positive effects have worn off. Once the short-term increase in brain efficiency and the pleasure of the endorphins have worn off, the negative side effects take over. Muscle tension, anxiety, unfounded fears, and even headaches are common.

If you're going to use caffeine to boost neurotransmission, I recommend that you use smaller amounts. Don't drink more than two cups of coffee per day, or substitute black tea for coffee. Black tea, as you are probably well aware, does not have anywhere near the side effects that coffee does. (See chapter 6 for a complete list of caffeine-containing foods.)

PROTEIN FOR POWER LUNCHES

You've got an important lunch meeting with aggressive and powerful people, and there's a lot on the line. You arrive at the restaurant a little agitated and slightly low. You need a boost. The waiter hands you the menu, which you scan in a perfunctory way, thinking instead about what you're going to say, how you should approach these people, and worrying about the outcome of your performance. Stop thinking about your presentation for a moment and concentrate on the menu. You may not realize it, but the most important assistance you can get at this point comes not from your colleagues or your competitors, but from your waiter.

Here's the best brain chemistry strategy for your business lunch, or any business meeting for which you need rapid neurotransmission. First, order coffee or tea to instantly speed up neurotransmission. Second, order broiled fish, no butter, no dairy-based dressing. All you need is about three ounces of a protein food—the size of a deck of cards—to trigger sufficient dopamine and norepinephrine to make you more alert, keen of mind, and assertive. By declining the butter or dairy-based dressing, you have avoided the fat that would make your brain and body sluggish. You have also avoided the carbohydrate that is in dairy foods, which would stimulate a relaxation response. Eat your salad last.

Avoid alcohol, an extreme carbohydrate that will trigger relaxation and even sleepiness. Also, forgo the rolls, breadsticks, pasta, and dessert—all carbohydrate foods that will make you focused, but also more relaxed and passive. As for the salad greens, they are low in carbohydrate—greens are rich in minerals, vitamins, and fiber, but low in starch—and their effect on your brain chemistry will be essentially neutral.

When you get home at night and want to relax, bring on the carbohydrates—pasta and a little dessert, if you like. But if you're jousting with the competition during the day and want to be alert, protein is your best bet.

Method 2: The Long-Term Approach to Peak Performance

Your brain makes up approximately 2 percent of your total body weight, yet it uses about 25 percent of all the oxygen you take in. If your brain is deprived of oxygen for four minutes or more, you will suffer significant brain damage. If you are deprived of oxygen for seven minutes, you'll be brain dead, if not physically dead. Your brain requires that much oxygen because it does so much work. The brain governs and monitors every action taking place within your body, including all conscious and autonomic functions. It is the physical tool of your consciousness: Every thought, emotion, and sensation coming from all five of your senses is processed by your brain. Your brain is continually working, even while you sleep.

All this work requires an enormous amount of energy, and energy requires oxygen. Oxygen is used by your cells — including your brain cells — to burn fuel. Fuel comes in the form of glucose, or blood sugar. Oxygen is carried to your brain and body cells by red blood cells that travel through your bloodstream. Through a highly complex chemical reaction, glucose combines with heat and oxygen to oxidize within the cell, creating energy. That energy is stored in your body cells and brain as adenosine triphosphate, or ATP.

Anything that diminishes the amount of oxygen flowing to the brain affects the brain's capacity to use energy and function. As blood flow to the brain is slowed, oxygen is not available in the abundance that the brain requires. In addition, carbon dioxide levels build. As a result, the brain becomes less efficient, tired, and sluggish.

The main factors that control the flow of oxygen to the brain — and all other organs in the body — are diet and exercise. Specifically, the higher the fat and cholesterol content of the diet, the less oxygen will be present in your blood, which means that less oxygen will get to your brain. Oxygen is carried in the blood by red blood cells, which are shaped like donuts with a little opening in the middle of each cell. Fat and cholesterol cause your red blood cells to become sticky and adhere to one another, much like a roll of coins. When this happens, their oxygen-carrying capacity is significantly reduced. The result is that less oxygen is brought to cells throughout the body, including the brain. Also, whenever red cells stick together, they can no longer squeeze through many of the smaller capillaries that provide blood to cells throughout the body, including the brain. Thus fat and cholesterol prevent the red blood cells from carrying optimal amounts of oxygen, and keep the blood and oxygen from going where it normally must go. Both effects reduce the amount of blood that gets to your brain, which makes the brain tired and sluggish and slows neurotransmission. We've all experienced the effects of such clumping. Think back to the last time you had a rich, heavy meal. I'm willing to bet that after the meal you couldn't think very well and wanted desperately to take a nap.

When we persist in eating foods rich in fat and cholesterol, over time we drive the fat content of our blood up, which limits the amount of oxygen that gets to the brain. When fat and cholesterol levels remain high, they cause an underlying disease called atherosclerosis, which is the narrowing of arteries that bring oxygen-enriched blood to organs. Atherosclerosis is the primary cause of most heart attacks and strokes that occur in the United States and the Western world. Atherosclerosis, of course, limits the amount of blood getting to the brain. In time, it can diminish oxygen flow to the brain, slow neurotransmission, cause senility, and eventually cause a stroke.

DIET AND EXERCISE

Fortunately, you can easily increase the amount of oxygen getting to your brain by lowering the fat and cholesterol content of your diet. Just by eating a diet that is based on whole grains, fresh vegetables, fruit, and low-fat animal products, you can dramatically improve your mental acuity within as little as two weeks.

Nathan Pritikin, the pioneering scientist who created the Pritikin program for diet and exercise, used to give people a simple math test when they began his program at the Pritikin Longevity Center in

Santa Monica, California. The questions on the math test were all very easy—$2 \times 5 = ?$; $25 \times 7 = ?$; $45 \times 4 = ?$, for example. He'd ask people to solve as many of these simple mathematical equations as they could in, say, 60 seconds. Pritikin would administer the same test to the same people after they had been at the Longevity Center for four weeks. The results were remarkable. After four weeks of healthful eating, everyone's test scores went up dramatically. They could solve more problems in less time. Everyone got smarter because their brains functioned more efficiently on the healthy regimen.

Of course, exercise also increases blood flow throughout the body and this, in turn, will increase the oxygen content of brain cells, thus causing neurotransmission to speed up. You do not have to do a lot of exercise to increase mental acuity or overall fitness. Walking three or four times a week for at least twenty minutes a session will increase your fitness and pump more blood and oxygen to your brain.

Take Care of Your Brain, So It Can Take Care of You

There are at least two ways you can improve the gas mileage of your car. The first is simply to drive at a steady pace, say fifty miles an hour. This keeps a consistent flow of fuel going to your car's motor, and therefore maintains the motor at a steady rpm, which in turn gives you maximum gas mileage. The second way is to tune up your car's motor so that it runs more efficiently.

Brain chemistry works in a similar fashion. You can maintain or alter your moods by providing a steady flow of neurotransmitters, or you can increase the efficiency with which your brain works. As we've seen, moods depend on the availability of certain neurotransmitters inside your brain. The more you have of certain neurotransmitters— say dopamine or serotonin—the more your mood state will lean in one direction or another. If you want to improve your mood, you can change the amount of neurotransmitter available.

You can also increase oxygen to your brain simply by lowering fat and cholesterol and eating foods high in complex carbohydrates. This will give you long-lasting energy and a clear mind.

Both slow and fast neurotransmission have their advantages and disadvantages. The danger occurs when we are out of balance and have no control over how fast or slow we are going. In the next chapter, we'll look at healthy and healing diets for Satiation and Arousal personalities that provide long-term peak performance.

6

Foods for a
Healthy Brain and
a Healthy Body

The Three Food Zones

The next two chapters discuss peak performance diets for both Satiation and Arousal personalities. This chapter includes general guidelines as well as lists of foods that boost serotonin and those that increase dopamine and norepinephrine. In chapter 7, the foods are organized into diets for Satiation and Arousal personalities. Please read both chapters carefully.

First, however, I want you to understand which foods will boost serotonin and which ones will increase dopamine and norepinephrine — and at the same time enhance your overall health. I want you to know the effects of individual foods on your brain chemistry *and* on your overall health.

Therefore I have divided foods into three zones from which you can choose: the Healthy Zone, the Occasional Zone, and the Red Zone. No matter whether you are a Satiation or an Arousal personality, you can choose your diet from this basic pool of foods. Each of the three zones contains both serotonin boosters and dopamine and norepinephrine boosters. You can choose health-enhancing serotonin boosters or health-enhancing dopamine boosters from the Healthy Zone. You can choose foods that will boost either serotonin or dopamine from the Occasional Zone, and you can choose both kinds of neurochemical boosters from the Red Zone.

How to Approach Your New Performance Diet

You can approach the peak-performance programs below in one of two ways. You can choose the appropriate healing lifestyle for you and adopt it as a fundamental part of your everyday life; or you can use your program as a form of medication—which is to say, as a set of foods and exercises that you adopt whenever the symptoms of your imbalance arise. In the latter case, you would follow the recommendations for as long as your symptoms persist.

It all depends on what you want to accomplish. If you adopt the program as a way of life, you will gradually change your baseline neurochemistry and free yourself from any negative symptoms of your underlying imbalance. You will not be subjected to the enormous swings in mood and mental functioning that you may be enduring now. Instead, you will establish a far more stable foundation for your life. The first approach, therefore, is a new way of living. It will give you the greatest rewards over time.

On the other hand, change can be difficult, and sometimes the best approach is to make changes incrementally. You may want to try to adopt aspects of the program now, and gradually increase your compliance as you learn to prepare and enjoy some of the new foods on the diet and incorporate some of the exercises into your lifestyle.

Hanging Tough During Your Transition Period

Giving up certain foods that you now enjoy may be difficult, especially since your brain rewards you for eating them. Also, as described
in our earlier discussion of adenylate cyclase, brain chemistry will, at
least for a transition period, adjust itself somewhat to sustain what it
considers normal. During that time, you will likely experience improvements of your moods and mental functioning, but there will also
be times when the old moods and old ways of seeing life will reassert
themselves. It's as if there is a struggle between the new way of living
and the old, a struggle between the light and the dark.

Don't become discouraged. Gradually, your new baseline will be
established, and with it a new mental and emotional stability will
form. Remember, it took you many years to establish your current
baseline neurochemistry. Suddenly, you're changing it—and changing it rapidly. Naturally, there will be periods in which the old moods
and mental states surface. However, if you follow the appropriate program for you, making adjustments to suit your own needs, these dark
moods or times of dull mental functioning should pass quickly.

If you are feeling depressed, you can (1) increase serotonin by increasing foods rich in carbohydrates, preferably complex carbohydrates (see the list below); and (2) follow the exercises appropriate for
your condition (described in chapter 8). In a short while, your moods
will be swinging up again.

If you're feeling anxious, you can lower your dopamine and norepinephrine by (1) decreasing foods rich in protein; and (2) doing
some vigorous exercise, which will burn up a lot of dopamine and restore your peace of mind.

As much as possible, do not feed your depression by indulging
too much in simple sugars or alcohol. Both will only make the condition worse. Conversely, don't feed your anxiety by drinking too much
coffee and eating protein-rich foods. They'll only make the anxiety
worse.

Substitutions and Counterbalancing Foods

In order to make this adjustment as smooth and as comfortable as possible, you should gradually decrease any unhealthy foods you are currently using, and begin to use healthy substitutions and eat counterbalancing foods. *Substitutions* are foods that provide an effect that is similar to the food you may be giving up. *Counterbalancing foods* promote the opposite set of neurotransmitters, which will balance your overall brain chemistry.

For example, if you are exceedingly high in dopamine and want to control your anxiety, you may want to eat less red meat and whole eggs, or give up both entirely. At the same time, you still want some protein in your diet to maintain a certain level of brain chemistry and function. In that case, you can substitute fish or poultry—both high-protein foods—as well as vegetable proteins, such as beans, tofu, and tempeh (all described below).

You should also eat fish and poultry less frequently than you formerly ate red meat or eggs. In the past, you may have eaten red meat and eggs every day, or even two or three times per day. Now you may want to eat fish or chicken three times a week, and eventually drop that down to twice a week. By reducing or eliminating red meat and eggs, and eating fish or poultry two or three times a week, you will decrease your dopamine and norepinephrine levels and significantly lower your anxiety.

Meanwhile, you will also want to eat counterbalancing foods that promote the opposite neurotransmitter, and thus establish a greater balance within your brain chemistry. For example, if you are anxious you will want to increase your intake of carbohydrates—from grains such as brown rice, wheat, wheat bread; noodles; vegetables; and fruit—all of which will increase brain levels of serotonin and enhance your sense of self-esteem and well-being and your ability to relax and concentrate. This alone will decrease anxiety and stress.

Where Will I Get My Protein?

Protein is used by the body for the creation of hormones and for cell replacement and repair. In order to meet and exceed all of the body's requirements for protein, an adult must eat 20 grams of protein per day, which amounts to about two-thirds of an ounce. You can get that much protein and more per day by just eating your fill of potatoes.

No one is suggesting that you eat only potatoes (which, by the way, are an otherwise wonderful serotonin booster). The point I'm making is that as long as you eat a diet based largely on whole foods — such as whole, unrefined grains, vegetables, beans, and fruit—*you cannot become deficient in protein, even if the diet is composed entirely of vegetables.* Most whole, unrefined vegetable foods contain complete protein. In fact, no nutritionist can create a diet made up of whole vegetable foods that is inadequate in protein, even for a child. I am not recommending vegetarianism per se, although I have nothing but positive things to say about such diets as long as they are nutritionally adequate. Nevertheless, I encourage you to eat healthful amounts of animal foods regularly, if you'd like, and to adjust those amounts to suit your brain chemistry and overall health.

Most Americans eat far too much protein. Science has demonstrated that excess protein is linked to osteoporosis, kidney disorders, and several types of cancer. The U.S. Surgeon General, along with the National Academy of Sciences and other prestigious scientific groups, has encouraged Americans to reduce their intake of protein-rich foods, and especially to reduce consumption of animal protein. All suggested programs fall within the health recommendations of these leading health authorities. The reason is simple: Foods that are rich in protein are also rich in fat, and usually they're rich in cholesterol. Many of the animal sources of protein—red meat, eggs, and many dairy products—are high-fat foods. Some exceptions to this are fish and the white meat of poultry. (I have provided a chart for you to compare the protein and fat content of foods, below.) All animal foods have cholesterol, as well.

All of this means that if you view your diet only from the serotonin-dopamine axis, you might be led to believe that the only effect of high consumption of animal foods is a high dopamine content, but that would not be true. You'd also increase your risk of heart disease, cancer, adult-onset diabetes, and other serious disorders.

By following these programs, you can lower the fat and cholesterol content of your diet and significantly lower your blood cholesterol, which will help protect you from heart disease, cancer, and other life-threatening illnesses. In other words, you'll feel good in both body and mind.

Everyone Needs Serotonin

All of us need serotonin. It boosts our sense of well-being, our self-esteem, and our ability to concentrate, and makes it possible for us to enjoy deep and restful sleep. Studies have shown that people with low serotonin are more prone to violence, including self-inflicted violence. Other research has shown that when animals and people rise in status, their serotonin levels also increase. As more and more people turn to drugs like Prozac and Zoloft—both serotonin boosters—it becomes clear that our society is being divided among those who are able to maintain normal serotonin and those who are not.

We need dopamine and norepinephrine as well; but we must remember that throughout our long history, humans have subsisted mostly on whole grains, vegetables, and fruits, eating animal products in smaller quantities. Indeed, in most traditional cultures even today, people eat far more vegetable foods—grains, beans, greens, and fruit—than animal products. Their serotonin levels are probably higher than ours, too. By eating appropriately from the lists offered below, anyone can increase serotonin while lowering, maintaining, or raising dopamine and norepinephrine, as appropriate for your type.

Three Zones for Healthy Choices

No matter what type you are, you can choose the foods you eat from the three groups described below, but you should try to derive most of your diet from the *Healthy Zone*. The *Occasional Zone* is composed of foods that can give you an immediate lift and which can be eaten occasionally without negative side effects (unless you have a particular sensitivity to one or another of these foods). The *Red Zone* contains foods that have striking effects on brain chemistry, but have negative side effects on health.

In general, I recommend that you eat only foods from the first two categories. If you do eat foods in the Red Zone, use moderation or eat them when you are feasting, such as on holidays, birthdays, and days of celebration. If you reserve these foods for special occasions, you can avoid their negative health effects.

1. The Healthy Zone

Serotonin Boosters

WHOLE GRAINS

Everyone wants to have energy, endurance, and stamina. Your best source of energy is from complex carbohydrates, which are found most abundantly in whole grains.

Whole grains—grains that have not been stripped of their nutrition by the refining process—provide the greatest assortment of nutrition in the food supply. Whole grains contain complex carbohydrates, protein, minerals, vitamins (especially vitamin E), and fiber. Harvard University agronomist professor Paul C. Manglesdorf said that a

The Three Food Zones

	Healthy Zone	Occasional Zone	Red Zone
SEROTONIN BOOSTERS	whole grains	cereals with milk	simple sugars
	flour products	waffles or pancakes	alcohol
	squashes		
	root vegetables	potato chips	
	whole-grain snacks and desserts	corn chips	
	fruit-sweetened candies	crackers and cheese	
	popcorn without added fats		
	fruit juice		
NEUTRAL FOODS	green, yellow, orange, and leafy vegetables		
	fruit		
	water		
DOPAMINE AND NOREPINEPHRINE BOOSTERS	fish and seafood	chicken	eggs
	beans, legumes, and bean products	turkey	red meat
	seeds and nuts	coffee	whole-milk dairy products
	black or green tea	non-fat or low-fat milk	

whole-grain cereal, if its food values are not destroyed by the over-refining of modern processing methods, comes closer than any other plant product to providing an adequate diet.

Complex carbohydrates are long chains of sugar molecules that are broken down by saliva and enzymes in your intestines. These long chains of sugars are then made available to your bloodstream in a constant, methodical way, as if your body were feeding itself over several hours. Contrast these with simple carbohydrates, which come in the form of white, refined sugars that are absorbed into the bloodstream the minute you put them into your mouth. Within minutes, they dramatically raise your blood sugar levels and are then quickly burned. They provide a quick burst of energy but are quickly spent, leaving you without much available fuel. The result is that you feel tired, listless, moody, and anxious, a condition referred to as hypoglycemia.

Whole grains include: brown rice, barley, millet, wheat, corn, amaranth, sweet rice, wild rice, teff, quinoa, and oats. In addition, you can try cracked grains, which can be prepared in minutes and provide whole-grain nutrition. These include bulgar (or cracked wheat), tabouli, Wheatena, and couscous.

FLOUR PRODUCTS

When whole grains are milled into flour for bread, they are broken up into tiny bits, which allows them to be absorbed more rapidly by the small intestine. This also increases the speed with which carbohydrates enter the bloodstream, so they boost brain levels of serotonin levels quickly.

Flour products include: whole-grain breads of all kinds; and whole-grain chapatis, bagels, tortillas, tacos, and pasta.

SQUASH AND PUMPKIN

Squashes of all kinds, baked or boiled, are sweet, delicious serotonin boosters.

Squashes include: acorn squash, butternut squash, pumpkin, hakkaido pumpkin, hubbard squash, yellow squash, and zucchini.

ROOT VEGETABLES

A rich source of carbohydrates, fiber, and many important vitamins and minerals, root vegetables are a wonderful and delicious part of any meal. Baked potatoes, of course, are an American staple. Yams and sweet potatoes are rich in beta carotene, an immune booster and cancer fighter. Roots are wonderful as root stews, in salads, and as side dishes. And all the roots are great serotonin boosters.

Root vegetables include: potatoes, sweet potatoes, carrots, onions, rutabagas, turnips, ginger, burdock, red radish, daikon radish, celery, and lotus root.

SNACKS AND DESSERTS

Desserts that boost serotonin levels and are good for you are generally made with whole grains and without refined sugar.

Snacks and desserts include: whole-grain cookies sweetened with apple juice or rice syrup; whole-grain crackers; boxed cereals eaten dry, or with apple juice, rice milk, or soy milk instead of milk; rice cakes with jam or rice syrup; cakes and pastries made with whole-grain flour and sweetened with fruit juice, rice syrup, barley malt, and other natural sweeteners; candies made from fruit juice and other natural ingredients; popcorn without added fats; whole-grain raisin bread; corn chips or pinta chips made from organically grown corn or beans and vegetable oils.

Neutral Foods

GREEN, YELLOW, ORANGE, AND LEAFY VEGETABLES

Vegetables are among the richest sources of vitamins and minerals in the entire food supply. This is why green, red, orange, and leafy vegetables have a neutral effect on brain chemistry in the short term, but an indirect serotonin-boosting effect in the longer term. A couple of hours after a protein meal is digested and the amino acid tyrosine is fully spent, these vegetables often encourage the brain to utilize the leftover tryptophan, the precursor of serotonin, that is also found in animal foods.

Remember, animal foods do contain tryptophan, but they contain so many other amino acids that very little of the tryptophan actually gets on the transport system that allows amino acids to pass through the blood-brain barrier and into the brain tissue. Hence the net effect of high-protein foods, especially animal foods, is to raise the blood levels of tyrosine and thus increase dopamine and norepinephrine in your brain. A few hours after a protein meal, these neurochemicals are burned up and a new flow of amino acids is sought by the brain.

Since vegetables are neutral, they have little or no effect on brain chemistry. Instead, the brain draws from the blood the leftover tryptophan that was not used originally when the animal foods were eaten. Thus a few hours after that protein meal was consumed, the leftover tryptophan is consumed and serotonin is increased.

Despite their small effects on brain chemistry, vegetables promote overall health, which boosts brain efficiency. I encourage you to eat them as a way of preventing disease and promoting good health.

The variety of the vegetable kingdom is virtually limitless. Here's a sample: asparagus, artichokes, beets, beet greens, bamboo shoots, Chinese cabbage, broccoli, collard greens, Brussels sprouts, cabbage, dandelion root, daikon radish, green peas, cucumber, dandelion greens, lotus root, endive, mushrooms (of all types), escarole, okra, kale, kohlrabi, leeks, lettuce (preferably dark green or red lettuce), mustard greens, scallions, string beans, sprouts, Swiss chard, watercress.

Among the most nutritious vegetables are: broccoli, cabbage, collard greens, mustard greens, and watercress.

FRUIT

Fruit has a neutral effect on brain chemistry because fructose must be converted to glucose in the small intestine. It takes too much time for the sugar in fruit to be converted to glucose, which would promote serotonin production in the brain. Fruit boosts immune function, promotes intestinal health (thanks to its high fiber content), and is loaded with cancer-preventing nutrients. Eat a piece of fruit a day, and your entire body will thank you.

WATER

Water is still the drink the body needs the most. It keeps you alive, but has a neutral effect on brain chemistry.

Dopamine and Norepinephrine Boosters

FISH AND SEAFOOD

Many fish are not only the most protein-rich foods on the planet, but they're also low in fat. This means that fish will provide a fast dopamine and norepinephrine boost but will not raise your blood cholesterol level substantially or block oxygen from the brain.

The healthiest fish available include: cod, haddock, flounder, salmon, scrod, snapper, swordfish, trout, tuna, sea bass, and bass; shrimp, scallops, and lobster (with low to moderate amounts of cholesterol, but generally low in fat); canned fish, including tuna packed in water; sardines packed in water; pickled herring; anchovies.

BEANS, LEGUMES, AND BEAN PRODUCTS

Beans are a rich source of protein and thus a dopamine and norepinephrine booster. There are also several very healthful and protein-rich bean products, such as tofu, tempeh, and natto. Tofu is widely available in most supermarkets and natural foods stores. Tempeh is a fermented bean product, much like cheese, that can be fried as a patty, like a hamburger, or used in soups. Natto is a fermented soybean condiment often used in Asia on rice and other grains.

Beans include: adzuki beans, black-eyed peas, black beans, chickpeas, kidney beans, lima beans, lentils, navy beans, pinto beans, soybeans (including yellow and black soybeans).

Bean products include: tofu, tempeh, and natto.

SNACKS

Many seeds and nuts are dopamine and norepinephrine boosters.

Seeds and nuts include: sunflower, pumpkin, and sesame seeds; almonds, cashews, walnuts, Brazil nuts, and others.

2. The Occasional Zone

Serotonin Boosters

FRUIT JUICE

Fruit juice is a serotonin booster and is very healthful when consumed in moderate amounts. Many varieties do contain simple sugars, however, which can adversely affect blood sugar, especially for sensitive people.

Dopamine and Norepinephrine Boosters

CHICKEN

Chicken is relatively low in fat and high in protein. Try to buy the range-fed and organically grown type. Factory-raised chicken can become contaminated by steroids, antibiotics, and other chemicals. These chickens often live under dirty and highly toxic conditions as well, which makes salmonella poisoning all too common.

You should also avoid eating the skin of the chicken, which is where you'll find much of the fat. Fat cells are the sites where all animals store the toxic substances they ingest (humans do the same); so chicken skin is not only rich in fat, but the most likely place where poisons will be located. I recommend that you always remove the skin of the chicken before eating the meat.

My recommendation: As long as the chicken is clean, it can be a healthful food and a good dopamine and norepinephrine booster.

TURKEY

Many people think that turkey is a serotonin booster because it is rich in tryptophan, the precursor of serotonin. In fact, the high protein content of turkey floods the blood with tyrosine as well as tryptophan, creating a competition for transport beyond the blood-brain barrier. More tyrosine than tryptophan ends up getting into the brain, so the net effect of turkey is to raise dopamine and norepinephrine levels.

COFFEE

Coffee is a major and almost instantaneous dopamine and norepinephrine booster. There is scant evidence that coffee is related to any serious illness, though some studies link high doses of coffee with fibrocystic breast disease and bladder cancer. Limit coffee to two cups per day, if you choose to drink it.

BLACK OR GREEN TEA

Both black tea and green tea contain about 45 milligrams of caffeine. They are rich in antioxidants and other immune-boosting and cancer-fighting nutrients.

LOW-FAT OR NON-FAT MILK

Milk contains both protein and carbohydrate, and so will boost levels of both dopamine-norepinephrine and serotonin. Use only non-fat or low-fat milk to avoid fat.

3. The Red Zone

The Red Zone foods have dramatic effects on brain chemistry, and consequently are often abused. Some of these foods, such as refined sugars and alcohol, cause impressive increases in serotonin levels. Others, such as red meat and eggs, promote dopamine and norepinephrine. According to the U.S. Surgeon General, Americans eat too much red meat and consume too many eggs. There is too much alcohol abuse in the United States and we probably eat far too much sugar. We eat these foods in excess because they affect us in ways that we enjoy, or feel we need. In other words, they give us rewards. Nevertheless, these same foods cause the death of millions each year, and debilitate many millions more.

Rather than judge ourselves negatively for such overindulgence, we should recognize that the foods in the Red Zone are powerful and have extreme effects on both brain chemistry and health. Consequently, if we choose to eat these foods or drink alcohol, we should do so prudently and with moderation.

To give you an idea of why I have chosen to place some of these foods in the Red Zone—to be eaten or drunk in moderation or reserved for feasts—I have provided a chart that reveals the protein and fat content of certain foods. Some foods from the Healthy and Occasional Zones are included here as a means of comparison.

Fat is perhaps the strongest toxin in the food supply. It is responsible for more illness and deaths due to heart disease and cancer each year than any other nutrient or environmental poison. Many people abuse high-fat foods, in part because they provide a dopamine or norepinephrine boost.

I have also included in this chart the caffeine content of certain foods, including coffee, tea, and chocolate. Caffeine, a big arousal booster, is one of the last legal addictions; like its opposite number, alcohol, it is a substance that creates satiation.

Serotonin Boosters

These foods will boost serotonin levels, but will likely have adverse effects on blood sugar levels, causing mineral losses, hypoglycemia, hyperglycemia, and high triglyceride levels.

SIMPLE SUGARS

These sweeteners are commonly found in cakes, pastries, ice cream, donuts, and chocolates. Take note: Artificial sweeteners, many of which are made from proteins, may *decrease* brain serotonin levels. There is no need to use saccharin, aspartame, or other artificial sweeteners in your diet.

Simple sugars include: white sugar, brown sugar, fructose, honey, molasses, and corn sweeteners.

ALCOHOL

Alcohol is a concentrated refined carbohydrate and a big serotonin booster. Alcohol kills brain cells and impairs all mental

Percentage of Calories Derived from Protein and Fat

	Protein	Fat

Red Meat

Red meat includes beef, lamb, veal, venison, pork, and all processed meats (such as frankfurters and sausage). Red meats are rich in protein, as well as rich in fat. (They often contain high levels of steroids, antibiotics, and other chemicals that may have harmful side effects, including on brain chemistry.)

		Protein	Fat
BEEF	Boneless chuck, lean (with fat removed)	32%	68%
	Ground beef (hamburger)	34%	65%
	Corned beef	25%	74%
	T-bone steak (broiled)	16%	82%
	Veal, rib roast	36%	61%
LAMB	Leg	32%	66%
	Loin or lamb chops	22%	76%
PORK	Ham	21%	78%
	Pork chops, with bone	23%	75%
	Spareribs	16%	83%

Poultry

		Protein	Fat
CHICKEN	White meat without skin (most of the fat in chicken is located in the skin)	76%	18%
	Dark meat without skin	64%	32%
	Fried chicken and giblets	49%	43%
	Eggs, raw whole	33%	65%
	Egg whites	85%	7%
TURKEY	Roasted	41%	56%

Fish and Seafood

	Protein	Fat
Cod	89%	8%
Flounder (baked with butter or margarine; far less fat if broiled)	59%	37%
Mackerel	37%	60%
Sturgeon	63%	32%
Tuna (canned in oil)	34%	64%
Tuna (canned in water)	88%	56%
Lobster	79%	14%
Shrimp (fried)	84%	8%
Scallops, steamed	83%	11%

Dairy Products

	Protein	Fat
Whole milk	21%	49%
Low-fat milk (2%)	28%	31%
Skim milk	41%	2%
Cheddar cheese	25%	73%
Swiss cheese	30%	68%
Cottage cheese, whole	51%	36%
Cottage cheese, low-fat	79%	3%

Note: Because protein and fat are only two components of food, which also contains vitamins, minerals, carbohydrates, and, in the case of vegetables, fiber, some percentages given here do not add up to 100 percent.

functioning. There is evidence that it also decreases the body's own ability to produce serotonin.

Dopamine and Norepinephrine Boosters

These foods will boost dopamine and norepinephrine but will have significant side effects on health because of their fat and cholesterol content.

EGGS AND RED MEAT

The diets for Arousal types 1 and 2 in chapter 7 list the amounts of protein and fat in commonly consumed meats.

WHOLE-MILK DAIRY PRODUCTS

Dairy products, such as whole milk, cheeses, and yogurt, are a mixed bag when it comes to brain chemistry. They are high in protein, but contain carbohydrates as well. In fact, dairy products are the only animal food that contains both protein and carbohydrates. The reason they contain both is that dairy foods are actually mother's milk from the cow, designed to feed newborn cows the basic ingredients they need for life. The protein content of cow's milk is quite different from that of human mother's milk. Cow's milk, which has an average protein content of 2.4 grams per 100 milliliters of milk, has twice the protein of human milk, which contains 1.2 grams per 100 milliliters of milk. This difference in protein is necessary because cows grow faster and bigger than humans do—it takes a cow forty-seven days to double its birth weight; humans require 180 days. Whole cow's milk is also loaded with fat.

Because of the protein, carbohydrate, and fat content, cow's milk will have a neutral effect on brain chemistry for many, and a weakening effect for some.

Now you know the general effects of foods on brain chemistry and overall health, and should be able to choose wisely and judiciously. In the next chapter, you'll find diets designed specifically for Satiation and Arousal personalities.

7

Peak-Performance
Diets for Satiation
and Arousal Personalities

You Are What You Eat

B y now, you should know whether you are a Satiation or Arousal personality. In this chapter, we'll further refine those categories into Satiation personalities 1 and 2 and Arousal personalities 1 and 2, and offer peak-performance diets for each. The vast majority of people, no matter how mild or severe their symptoms, will fall into one of these types. Read the descriptions given in this chapter to determine which personality best fits you and follow the diet given.

Once you have decided on a diet, you will have to monitor yourself to determine if the recommended amounts of carbohydrates or protein are adequate or excessive for your condition. You may want to slightly increase or decrease your protein intake beyond the amounts suggested. As long as you are eating the balanced diet described in each of the categories, such small increases or decreases will not adversely affect your health and may well improve your brain chemistry.

A good way to monitor yourself is to keep a journal of your daily eating and exercise habits. Keep track of what seems to affect you and how. This is especially helpful if you are chronically and significantly depressed or anxious. If you keep a record in this way, you will soon discover the specific unconscious eating and exercise behaviors that affect your moods, and you will be able to adjust them more easily.

Two slightly different diets are given for each type of personality, one for Satiation types and the other for Arousal types. You must determine which Satiation or Arousal type you are, based upon the descriptions given.

Peak-Performance Diets for Satiation Personalities

There are two general types of Satiation personalities, which I have called 1 and 2. Read the following descriptions to determine which you are, and then follow the diet designed specifically for your type.

Satiation Personality 1. These people enjoy satiation activities, are emotionally low, and may be mildly to significantly biochemically depressed. At the same time, they have plenty of energy to perform whatever tasks they are required to do, and consequently rarely let their emotional condition affect their work. Indeed, people in this category are usually introverted, but quite competent and often heavily relied on. They are seen by others as steady, reliable, and even indispensable, if a bit dour and sensitive. As personalities they attract little or no attention and consequently are often overlooked or taken for granted.

Neurochemically, they have low serotonin but normal levels of dopamine and norepinephrine. Therefore the performance program is designed to raise their serotonin levels to boost their sense of well-being and joy and to relieve depression.

Satiation Personality 2. These people are also emotionally low and may be mildly to significantly biochemically depressed, but they lack the energy, the will, or the drive to accomplish goals. These people are often chronically fatigued, and their depression is much more vegetative. They tend to sit for hours doing little more than watching television or staring into space.

The performance program for Satiation type 2 will raise serotonin to help relieve depression and will mildly elevate dopamine and norepinephrine levels to increase energy, creativity, and willpower. I say mildly elevate dopamine and norepinephrine because Satiation personalities typically dislike and feel stressed by an abundance of gas-pedal neurochemicals.

If you are a Satiation personality 2, monitor yourself to make sure that you are not getting anxious and overly stressed from eating too many high-protein foods that will raise your dopamine and norepinephrine levels and increase your anxiety. You may want to monitor your protein intake on a regular basis.

Diet for Satiation Personality 1

This program is intended for the person who is emotionally low or depressed, but has significant amounts of energy. It is designed to elevate serotonin levels without substantially decreasing dopamine and norepinephrine. The diet emphasizes carbohydrate foods, which boost serotonin levels, but includes smaller amounts of animal protein. It especially encourages complex carbohydrates from whole grains, vegetables, fruit, and fruit juices, rather than simple sugars and artificial sweeteners.

GENERAL GUIDELINES

1. Reduce or eliminate red meat and eggs.
2. Eliminate chocolate, coffee, and caffeine-containing soft-drinks.
3. Snack on a complex carbohydrate two hours after eating a high-protein meal (this snacking will help you get the necessary amino acids).
4. Don't increase your overall calories for the day.

FOODS THAT WILL BOOST SEROTONIN AND INCREASE DOPAMINE

- *Whole grains,* such as brown rice, barley, oats, millet, and others, boiled or pressure-cooked (serotonin boosters): once or twice a day.
- *Flour products,* such as whole-grain pasta, whole-wheat bread, corn tortillas (serotonin boosters): daily.
- *Leafy green and yellow vegetables,* such as collard greens, kale, mustard, broccoli, and others (serotonin boosters): daily.
- *Root vegetables,* such as carrots, onions, celery, parsnips, turnips, rutabaga, potatoes, and others (serotonin boosters): twice a week.
- *Squashes,* such as acorn, buttercup, summer, zucchini, and others (serotonin boosters): twice a week.
- *Fruit* (serotonin boosters): daily.
- *Dried fruits* (serotonin boosters): whenever desired.
- *Vegetable protein foods,* such as beans, tofu, tempeh, and others (dopamine and norepinephrine boosters): twice a week.
- *Chicken or fish,* such as cod, scrod, flounder, halibut, and other low-fat fish; and salmon, which provides omega polyunsaturated fats that lower blood cholesterol (dopamine and norepinephrine boosters): once or twice a week.

MEAL PLAN SUGGESTIONS

Breakfast suggestions (serotonin boosters):

- Whole-grain hot cereal, such as oatmeal. Add raisins if desired; use rice syrup, barley syrup, or maple syrup for a sweetener.
- Leftover grain from dinner, such as brown rice, reheated with a little extra water to make the grain wetter and easier to digest; sweeten with rice syrup.
- Wheatena, with or without raisins; sweeten with rice syrup or maple syrup.

- Dry cereals, preferably with no added sugar (puffed rice and other puffed whole grains, Wheaties, Cheerios, Raisin Bran, and many others). If you would like to avoid dairy products, eat dry or use apple juice, rice milk, or soy milk as a substitute for milk.
- Whole-grain toast with jam.
- Whole-grain muffins, such as whole-wheat or bran muffins.
- Whole-grain English muffins.
- Hash brown potatoes. Hash browns now come packaged and prepared; all you have to do is heat them and serve.
- Lightly steamed or sautéed vegetables.

Breakfast suggestions (dopamine and norepinephrine boosters):

- Any type of fish, or fish soup.
- Smoked salmon (lox).
- Sliced tofu on toast, with a few drops of tamari or soy sauce, or with balsamic vinegar and fresh grated ginger root.
- Black tea.
- Green tea.
- Coffee.
- Red Zone: If you eat eggs, try to limit them to two eggs per week.

Lunch suggestions (serotonin boosters):

- Leftover grain from dinner.
- Sandwiches composed of whole-grain bread, leafy green vegetables, salad, mustard, balsamic vinegar, olive oil.
- Pasta.
- Hash brown potatoes.
- Greens and mixed vegetable salad.

- Lightly steamed or sautéed vegetables.
- Vegetable soup, such as minestrone.
- Whole-grain burgers (veggieburgers), with a variety of toppings, on whole-grain bread or bun; available ready-made, just defrost and reheat before lunch.
- Whole-grain chapati sandwiches, made of brown rice and vegetables and wrapped in chapati (widely available in natural foods stores).

Lunch suggestions (dopamine and norepinephrine boosters):

- Tuna salad sandwich.
- Chicken or turkey salad sandwich.
- Fish sandwich.
- Fish (any type).
- Beans.
- Tofu hot dogs.
- Tacos with beans.
- Tortillas with beans.
- Bean chili.

Dinner suggestions (serotonin boosters):

- A whole grain, such as brown rice, wild rice, barley, millet (pressure-cooked or boiled), tabouli, and others; with any number of condiments.
- Vegetable or grain soup.
- Pasta, any one of a wide variety of noodles (but not egg noodles, which are loaded with protein) with marinara sauce or some other vegetable topping of your choice.
- Steamed or sautéed leafy green vegetable.
- Baked squash.

- A root vegetable, or vegetable medley that includes roots, mushrooms, and broccoli.
- Salad, with a variety of leafy greens, celery, carrot, cucumber.

Dinner suggestions (dopamine and norepinephrine boosters):

- Broiled fish, any type, any preparation desired.
- Chicken, turkey.
- Beans (see lunch).
- Bean burrito, taco, chapati.
- Tofu and tempeh.
- Tea, black or green, or decaffeinated.

Diet for Satiation Personality 2

This program is designed for people who are mildly to significantly depressed, but are also chronically fatigued and lack alertness, willpower, and healthy aggression.

When you have these symptoms you are suffering from low serotonin *and* low dopamine and norepinephrine, so this diet boosts all three neurotransmitters. In general, you should emphasize carbohydrate foods and eat moderate amounts of protein.

GENERAL GUIDELINES

Follow the program for Satiation personality 1, but strictly adhere to the following advice:

1. Avoid snacking on carbohydrates between meals. Do not eat any grain products, such as bread, crackers, pastries, or rice cakes, between meals.

2. Scrupulously avoid refined white sugar, especially in the morning. Substitute oatmeal, whole grains, whole-grain cereals, or toast.

3. Eat one high-protein dish per day, and monitor your protein in-take to see how much you can eat without causing anxiety. Choose your protein meal from the Healthy Zone.

4. Begin each day with a whole-grain dish. This includes oatmeal, leftover rice, toast (apply jam lightly). You may sweeten it with raisins, rice syrup, maple syrup, or barley malt.

5. Experiment by eating a protein food in the morning to see how it affects your energy levels and morning demeanor.

6. Include a high-protein dish for dinner to see how it affects you the following day.

MEAL PLAN SUGGESTIONS

Follow the diet for Satiation personality 1, but increase protein foods slightly. Here are some suggestions for increasing protein and thereby boosting dopamine and norepinephrine.

Breakfast suggestions:

• Four to five days per week, eat a whole grain or whole-grain flour product (such as whole-wheat toast).

• Two days per week, eat any type of fish, or fish soup; smoked salmon (lox); or sliced tofu on toast, with a few drops of tamari or soy sauce, or balsamic vinegar with grated ginger root.

• If you eat eggs, limit them to two a week.

• Drink black tea, green tea, decaffeinated tea, or coffee.

Lunch suggestions:

• Four days per week eat a whole-grain, vegetable, or flour product.

• Three days per week, eat any of the following: tuna salad sand-wich, chicken or turkey salad sandwich; fish sandwich; fish (any type); bean burrito; tofu hot dog; tacos with beans; tortillas with beans; bean chili.

• Daily: fruit; some naturally sweetened dessert when desired.

Dinner suggestions:

- Four or five days a week eat a dinner that includes some combination of the following—a whole grain or noodles as a main course; vegetables, potato, soup, and dessert.

- Three days per week, include any of the following in your dinner meal: fish, chicken, beans, tofu, or tempeh.

Peak-Performance Diets for Arousal Personalities

There are two general types of Arousal personalities, which I have called 1 and 2. Read the following descriptions to determine which you are, and then follow the diet designed specifically for your type.

Arousal Personality 1. Arousal personality 1 arises from low serotonin coupled with higher than comfortable levels of dopamine and norepinephrine. These people suffer from anxiety, restlessness, fear, or insecurities, coupled with mild to significant depression. The anxiety may be covering up the depression, which is only felt when the person tries to settle down and relax. Consequently, these people resist relaxation. Many hate to relax. The best option is to boost serotonin by increasing carbohydrates, lowering protein, and following the exercise program offered in chapter 8. The increase in carbohydrates consumption will displace some of the protein they are eating, so dopamine and norepinephrine will naturally come down.

Arousal Personality 2. These people are simply too high in dopamine and norepinephrine, causing anxiety, fear, and insecurity, and maybe even paranoia. In general, this type of imbalance is corrected by decreasing dopamine and norepinephrine levels, which will decrease anxiety and all the other characteristics associated with elevated gas-pedal neurochemicals.

Diet for Arousal Personality 1

This program is designed for Arousal types who are both anxious and depressed, conditions that can be remedied by increasing serotonin and decreasing the gas-pedal neurotransmitters. The diet increases carbohydrate-rich foods to raise serotonin and reduces protein to lower dopamine and norepinephrine. This is easily accomplished by increasing foods rich in complex carbohydrates, which will mean that you are essentially substituting carbohydrates for protein.

GENERAL GUIDELINES

1. Significantly increase all complex carbohydrate foods, such as whole-grain brown rice, oats, millet, barley, and buckwheat.
2. Significantly increase all whole-grain or milled pasta dishes, such as noodles, whole-grain breads, crackers, and other flour products.
3. Eliminate or significantly reduce all beef, luncheon meats, lamb, pork, pork products, and eggs.
4. Eliminate or significantly reduce all caffeinated beverages and foods containing caffeine, such as chocolate.
5. Significantly reduce or eliminate all hard cheeses and whole-milk products, such as cheddar cheese, Swiss cheese, and others.
6. Follow the exercise program outlined in chapter 8.

FOODS THAT WILL BOOST SEROTONIN

- Whole grains, such as brown rice, barley, oats, millet, and others, boiled or pressure-cooked: once or twice a day.
- Flour products, such as pasta, whole-wheat bread (sandwiches), or some other whole-grain flour food: daily.
- Leafy green or yellow vegetables, such as collard greens, kale, mustard greens, broccoli, and others: daily.
- Root vegetables, such as carrots, onion, celery, parsnips, turnips, rutabaga, and others: three times a week (carrots can be eaten daily).
- Squashes, such as acorn, buttercup, summer, zucchini, others, baked or boiled: twice a week.

- Fruit: daily.
- Dried fruits: whenever desired.

FOODS THAT MAINTAIN DOPAMINE AND NOREPINEPHRINE LEVELS

- Fish, low-fat fish such as cod, scrod, flounder, halibut, and others, and salmon, which provides omega polyunsaturated fats, which lower blood cholesterol: two or three times per week. (Ideally, you should lower your fish to once or twice a week after you have been on this program for several weeks and your baseline has begun to adjust to the lower levels of dopamine and norepinephrine.)
- Chicken: once a week (remove skin before eating).
- Vegetable protein foods, such as beans, tofu, and tempeh: once or twice a week.

MEAL PLAN SUGGESTIONS

Breakfast suggestions (serotonin boosters):

- Whole-grain hot cereal, such as oatmeal. Add raisins if desired; sweeten with rice syrup or maple syrup.
- Leftover grain from dinner, such as brown rice, reheated with a little extra water to make the grain wetter and easier to digest; sweeten with rice syrup.
- Wheatena, with or without raisins; sweeten with rice syrup or maple syrup.
- Dry cereals, preferably with no added sugar (puffed rice and other puffed whole grains, Wheaties, Cheerios, Raisin Bran, and many others). If you would like to avoid dairy products, eat dry or use apple juice, rice milk, or soy milk as a substitute for milk.
- Whole-grain toast with jam.
- Whole-grain muffins, such as whole-wheat or bran muffins.
- Whole-grain English muffins.

- Hash brown potatoes. Hash browns now come packaged and prepared; all you have to do is heat them and serve.
- Lightly steamed or sautéed vegetables.
- Fruit juice.

Breakfast suggestions (to maintain or boost dopamine and norepinephrine levels):

- Any type of fish, or fish soup.
- Smoked salmon (lox).
- Sliced tofu on toast, with a few drops of tamari or soy sauce, or balsamic vinegar with grated ginger root.
- Black or green tea.
- Coffee.

Lunch suggestions (serotonin boosters):

- Leftover grain from dinner.
- Sandwiches composed of whole-grain bread, leafy green vegetables (such as collard greens, kale, broccoli), salad, mustard, balsamic vinegar, olive oil.
- Pasta.
- Hash brown potatoes.
- Greens and mixed vegetable salad.
- Lightly steamed or sautéed vegetables.
- Vegetable soup, such as minestrone.
- Whole-grain burgers (veggieburgers), with a variety of toppings, on whole-grain bread or bun (available ready-made, just defrost and reheat before lunch).
- Wide variety of whole-grain chapati sandwiches, made of brown rice and vegetables and wrapped in chapati (widely available in natural foods stores).

Lunch suggestions (dopamine and norepinephrine boosters):

- Tuna salad sandwich.
- Chicken or turkey salad sandwich.
- Fish sandwich.
- Fish (any type).
- Beans.
- Tofu hot dogs.
- Tacos with beans.
- Tortillas with beans.
- Bean chili.

Dinner suggestions (serotonin boosters):

- A whole grain, such as brown rice, wild rice, barley, millet (pressure-cooked or boiled), tabouli, others; with any number of condiments.
- Vegetable or grain soup.
- Pasta, any one of a wide variety of noodles with marinara sauce or some other vegetable topping of your choice.
- Steamed or sautéed leafy green vegetable.
- Baked squash.
- A root vegetable, or vegetable medley that includes roots, mushrooms, and broccoli.
- Salad, with a variety of leafy greens, celery, carrot, cucumber.

Dinner suggestions (dopamine and norepinephrine boosters):

- Broiled fish, any type, any preparation desired.
- Chicken, turkey.
- Beans (see lunch).

- Bean burrito, taco, chapati.
- Tofu and tempeh.

Beverages:

- Tea, green or black.

Diet for Arousal Personality 2

This program is for people who are stressed, anxious, fearful, even paranoid. These people must lower dopamine and norepinephrine without lowering it so much that they become lethargic and chronically fatigued. Dopamine and norepinephrine levels are elevated by foods rich in protein and caffeine. Therefore, in order to reduce these two gas-pedal neurochemicals, you should reduce caffeine and foods high in protein.

GENERAL GUIDELINES

1. Reduce or eliminate all forms of red meat and eggs from your diet.
2. Rely on fish, chicken, beans, and tofu for your protein needs.
3. Decrease your intake of Healthy Zone and Occasional Zone animal foods to four times per week. After two to three weeks, reduce animal foods further again to three times per week. If symptoms persist, reduce animal foods to once or twice a week.
4. Include a whole-grain food or dish at every meal. This will boost your serotonin levels significantly. (See serotonin boosters under Satiation personality meal programs for suggestions.)
5. Snack on whole grains and foods made of whole-grain flour (rice cakes, cookies, popcorn, pastries, raisin bread, others).
6. Avoid nuts and seeds (they boost dopamine).
7. Eliminate or significantly reduce all caffeinated beverages and foods, such as chocolate.

8. Significantly reduce or eliminate all whole-milk products and hard cheeses, such as cheddar, Swiss, and others.

9. Follow the exercise program outlined in chapter 8.

FOODS THAT BOOST DOPAMINE AND NOREPINEPHRINE

- Fish, low-fat fish such as cod, scrod, flounder, and halibut, and salmon, which provides omega polyunsaturated fats, which lower blood cholesterol: two or three times per week. (Ideally, after you have been on the diet for several weeks and your baseline has begun to adjust to the lower levels of dopamine and norepinephrine, you should lower your fish intake to once or twice a week.)

- Chicken: once a week (remove skin before eating).

- Vegetable protein foods, such as beans, tofu, tempeh: once or twice a week.

- Whole grains, such as brown rice, barley, oats, millet, and others, boiled or pressure-cooked: once or twice a day.

- Flour products, such as pasta, whole-wheat bread (as in sandwiches), and others: daily.

- Leafy green or yellow vegetables, such as collard greens, kale, mustard greens, broccoli, and others: daily.

- Root vegetables, such as carrots, onion, celery, parsnips, turnip, rutabaga, others: twice a week.

- Squashes, such as acorn, buttercup, summer, zucchini, others: twice a week.

- Fruit: daily.

- Dried fruits: whenever desired.

Seeing the Forest *and* the Trees

Sometimes we can get so caught up in our own point of view that we can easily lose sight of the big picture. In the case of diet and health, the big picture is your overall good health. You can and should feel good in every way. By "good," I mean that you experience positive and buoyant moods, a clear and sharp mind, and a strong and healthy body that has an abundance of energy and is capable of preventing serious disease.

The best way to accomplish all of this is to make complex carbohydrate foods your basic physical and "feel-good" fuel. Protein foods should be your booster fuel—eat them when you need a lift, a spark, a boost to your personal and physical power.

In order to achieve this balance, make complex carbohydrates anywhere from 50 to 80 percent of your diet. Protein-rich foods should make up approximately 20 to 30 percent of your diet. The more protein foods you eat, however, the higher the percentage of your calories that will come from fat (the unavoidable by-product of those protein-rich foods). Nevertheless, as you bring protein into balance in your diet, you'll significantly reduce your fat and cholesterol consumption. The result will be that your mind will be clearer because your brain will be getting optimal amounts of oxygen, and your moods will be positive because you'll be getting plenty of tryptophan, which will raise your production of serotonin.

These dietary programs will help you change your neurochemistry toward a more balanced condition, and thus help you become emotionally happier and intellectually more alert. If you follow the dietary recommendations outlined in this chapter, you'll feel better in a matter of weeks. However, in order for the programs to have the desired effect, you will have to monitor yourself to determine two factors: Am I getting sufficient carbohydrates? and How much protein am I eating?

You can maintain the programs recommended and at the same time eat in restaurants and buy your food in food stores and natural foods stores. All it requires is a little planning and allowing yourself the time to adapt to a new way of eating. In no time, you will see—and feel—that the benefits far outweigh the effort.

There's more to this program than simply diet. Exercise, perceptions of life, and belief systems are also essential in achieving peace of mind. That is our goal—greater peace and tranquility of mind, body, and spirit. And with that, let's take the next step in our performance enhancement: adopting the right exercise program for mental and physical health.

8

Exercise Programs
for Satiation and
Arousal Personalities

Relaxing and Energizing Workouts

The effects of exercise on mood are dramatic and well documented. Studies have shown that exercise reduces depression, anxiety, and stress. It also significantly improves our outlook on life. One study that examined the effects of exercise on people being treated in a psychiatric hospital found that exercise significantly decreased depression and anxiety and increased a sense of accomplishment.

In addition to affecting serotonin and dopamine-norepinephrine levels, exercise also increases endorphins, the morphine-like compounds that provide a deep sense of well-being and a "natural high."

If you have high dopamine and norepinephrine levels, you're going to enjoy competitive sports and highly arousing aerobic exercise. Arousal types like the rough and tumble of competition and exertion. An Arousal personality who is forced to take low-impact aerobics, or walk, or meditate is liable to go a little batty—at least initially. If Arousal types practice low-impact aerobics or walking or meditation long enough, however, they will change their underlying baseline and begin to benefit enormously. But until that baseline changes, satiation practices will try their patience. Before long, Arousal types may be flying out of the room and looking desperately for their basketball or tennis racket.

On the other hand, a Satiation personality who must compete in a very intense athletic event most likely will become anxious and tense, especially if he particularly dislikes elevations in dopamine. So it's important to fit the right exercise program to the type of personality in question.

Exercise, no matter what your personality type, is very beneficial for overall good health. Aerobic exercise—exercise that increases the intake and utilization of oxygen—boosts the efficiency of the heart, causing the heart to pump more blood per beat and thus rest longer between beats. This, of course, takes the strain off the heart while it maintains your life.

You don't have to be an athlete to benefit from regular exercise. Studies show that your chances of living longer are increased dramatically if you simply walk three or more times per week for at least thirty minutes per walking session. Regular exercise boosts high-density lipoproteins (HDLs), the type of cholesterol that prevents heart attacks and strokes. Exercise also lowers your weight and blood pressure and reduces the risk of numerous degenerative diseases, including heart attack, stroke, cancer, and osteoporosis.

As with the diets offered in the previous chapter, you can choose your exercise program to establish a lifestyle or simply to increase or decrease the production of certain neurochemicals. One of the keys to success with any exercise program is that if it *feels* good, you'll keep at it.

Choosing the Right Exercise

Choose an exercise that you honestly enjoy doing. If you're looking for satiation, gentle walking and occasional hiking in nature are your best bet. Both can give you a low-exertion, health-enhancing workout that will boost serotonin levels. If you do not like competitive sports but want to improve your cardiovascular fitness, you can walk (with periodic increases in speed to increase heart rate), bicycle, run, or engage in water aerobics, aerobic dance, or some other aerobic exercise. If you enjoy sports, many games are highly aerobic and can be very satisfying. Here are some "exercise menus" from which to choose.

Exercises That Boost Serotonin

The following exercises will all boost your levels of serotonin. Done regularly, they will gently increase your level of fitness.

- Walking and strolling on a flat surface.
- Walking in nature (in a forest, along the beach, in a park).
- Bicycle riding on a flat surface with low exertion.
- Stretching.
- Low-impact aerobics.
- Any of the meditative Asian martial arts.
- Gentle weight lifting, with low weight.

Exercises That Temporarily Lower Dopamine and Norepinephrine and Increase Serotonin

The exercises in this category will initially arouse because they first increase dopamine and norepinephrine and then gradually burn off both. The net effect of these exercises, however, will be to temporarily lower dopamine levels and increase serotonin, promote cardiovascular fitness, and provide a sense of well-being and relaxation. In general, these include all highly aerobic exercises. However, weight lifting, an anaerobic exercise, also falls into this category. When an exercise is followed by a caution about being overly competitive, that means competitive to the point that your self-esteem depends on winning.

- Aerobic dance.
- Cross-country skiing.
- Jogging.
- Bicycling.
- Exercise bicycling.
- Stairmaster.
- Rowing machines.
- Nautilus.
- Treadmill machines.
- Hiking, especially uphill.
- Swimming.
- Water aerobics.
- High-exertion weight lifting.
- Basketball (as long as the player is not overly competitive).
- Tennis (as long as the player is not overly competitive).
- Racquetball (as long as the player is not overly competitive).

Exercises That Boost Dopamine and Norepinephrine and Raise Serotonin

The following exercises will raise dopamine and norepinephrine, then burn them off somewhat. If you take competition too seriously, however, they may keep both elevated to the point where your self-esteem depends on the outcome.

- All competitive sports, such as basketball, tennis, softball, racquetball, wrestling, competitive swimming, competitive weight lifting, and competitive track events (sprints, long-distance running, hurdles, javelin, shot-put, and others).

The Exercise Programs

In this section you will find four exercise programs geared to the four personality types: Satiation personalities 1 and 2 and Arousal personalities 1 and 2. As you did with diet in the previous chapter, determine which personality you are before choosing a program to follow.

Satiation type 1 has low serotonin but normal dopamine and norepinephrine. This Satiation type is emotionally low-key, and perhaps mildly to significantly depressed. The exercise program for this type is designed to increase serotonin.

Satiation type 2 has low serotonin and low dopamine and norepinephrine. This type is emotionally low, mildly to significantly depressed, and has low energy. Satiation type 2 is lethargic or chronically fatigued. The exercise program for this type is designed to boost serotonin (thus lessening depression) and increase the person's sense of strength and confidence (thanks to the fact that they increase dopamine and norepinephrine).

Arousal type 1 has low serotonin and high dopamine and norepinephrine, and thus is emotionally low (most are depressed) and at the same time anxious. The exercise program for this type is designed to increase serotonin and lower dopamine.

Arousal type 2 has normal serotonin but is excessively high in dopamine and norepinephrine and thus tends to be anxious, perhaps excessively so. This type is not particularly depressed, but is anxious and under stress. The exercise program for this type is designed to lower dopamine and norepinephrine.

THE LABELS "S" AND "A," AND A NOTE OF CAUTION

As you read the programs below, you will note that exercises that boost serotonin and satiation are labeled "S," while those that boost dopamine and norepinephrine, and thus heighten arousal, are labeled "A." An activity that creates relaxation and does not increase heart rate significantly is considered an "S" activity. An activity that increases heart rate and is associated with arousal is considered an "A" activity.

There are numerous choices within each of the "A" and "S" groups. You can walk or stretch or practice low-impact aerobics; all such exercises will be satiating and therefore fall under the "S" category. You can also jog, play tennis, do Nautilus, use a Stairmaster, or walk on a treadmill; all will be arousing and fall under the "A" group. Choose the exercises that most appeal to you. Again, the key to maintaining an exercise program is to do the things you enjoy. Make exercise fun.

An important note of caution: You should have a complete physical before you begin your exercise program. Also, if you feel more depressed or anxious after attempting any of the recommended exercises, please reread the program and consult your physician or health professional.

Exercise Program for Satiation Personality 1

This program is designed for the Satiation personality with low serotonin but normal dopamine and norepinephrine. These people have adequate to good energy, but are depressed. Therefore I recommend a combination of low-exertion, satiation exercises, along with exercises that will enhance cardiovascular fitness.

This program involves four days of satiation exercises, such as gentle walking, stretching, low-impact aerobics, and meditative martial arts, along with three days of noncompetitive aerobic exercise, such as bicycling, aerobic walking, or using a Nautilus, Stairmaster, or treadmill. You can play any of the competitive games, as long as you do not invest too much of your self-esteem in winning. Fortunately, people who fall into this type of Satiation personality tend to play the "inner game," which focuses on technique, skill development, and the enjoyment of the purity of the sport itself. If this is true for you, any competitive game that you enjoy can be a wonderful way to enhance your life and brain chemistry.

Here's your schedule:

Sunday: Satiation exercise, such as meditation, stretching, low-impact workouts, and other meditative exercises.

Monday: Arousal exercises. Anything aerobic or a competitive sport.

Tuesday: Satiation exercise.

Wednesday: Arousal routine.

Thursday: Satiation.

Friday: Arousal.

Saturday: Satiation.

DAILY SCHEDULE

	SUN	MON	TUE	WED	THUR	FRI	SAT
ROUTINE	S	A	S	A	S	A	S

If you feel stressed, perform an additional satiation activity. Follow your routine schedule to keep "in balance."

Exercise Program for Satiation Personality 2

If you are Satiation personality 2, you are emotionally low, perhaps depressed, and fatigued. Any type of exercise and activity will create mild to uncomfortable levels of dopamine and norepinephrine. Further, you probably dislike all situations and activities that create arousal, because they bring with them anxiety and often unbearable nervous tension. Therefore I recommend that you do seven days of satiation exercises, concentrating on meditation and meditative activities. The routines are noncardiovascular and nonaerobic. All should be relaxing. This will boost serotonin, relieve depression, and increase your sense of well-being.

Here's your schedule:

Sunday through Saturday: Morning meditation, followed by meditative exercises, such as walking, stretching, or low-impact aerobics.

DAILY SCHEDULE

	SUN	MON	TUE	WED	THUR	FRI	SAT
ROUTINE	S	S	S	S	S	S	S

Whenever you feel stressed, increase the cardiovascular aspect of your routine. Walk faster in spurts, and then resume your comfortable pace.

Exercise Program for Arousal Personality 1

If you are an Arousal personality 1, you have low serotonin and high dopamine and should avoid competitive athletics until you bring their neurochemistry into greater balance. People with this neurochemical profile tend to place their self-esteem into the outcome of the game. They lose perspective and stop enjoying the game for its sheer fun. Competitive situations tend to make such a neurochemical combination worse. Therefore I recommend that you avoid competitive games until you increase serotonin levels and feel ready to enjoy the "inner game," rather than focusing on defeating your opponent.

However, you need highly aerobic activities to work off excess dopamine and norepinephrine, and you also need a lot of satiation activities. The two must be combined, with satiation and serotonin boosters dominating the program. I recommend six days of satiation exercises, especially meditative, such as walking, low-impact aerobics, and the like, coupled with three days of noncompetitive highly aerobic exercises, including any of those listed above.

Use satiation exercises as bookends for your high-exertion aerobic exercise. Start out with a satiation exercise, such as walking or stretching; do your aerobic exercise; and finish with a satiation exercise.

Follow these guidelines:

- Perform five to ten minutes of satiation exercises to warm up, such as walking or stretching.
- Perform at least twenty minutes of arousing exercise, getting your heart rate up to at least 120 beats per minute.
- Conclude your aerobic workout with a ten- to fifteen-minute satiation exercise as your cooling-off period. Walking or stretching is ideal.

Here's your schedule:

DAILY SCHEDULE

	SUN	MON	TUE	WED	THUR	FRI	SAT
ROUTINE	S	S & A	S	S & A	S	S & A	S

When you feel stressed, perform an "A" activity. Follow your routine schedule to keep in balance.

Exercise Program for Arousal Personality 2

If you are Arousal personality 2 you have normal serotonin and high dopamine-norepinephrine, and you probably exercise quite a bit already. You probably especially enjoy competitive sports and love to get a good aerobic workout.

You must be cautioned not to overdo it. If you drive yourself too hard, you will raise your dopamine and norepinephrine beyond your tolerance levels and begin to experience excess anxiety and stress.

The best program for you is composed of three days per week of some arousing exercise, including competitive sports, especially if you enjoy a particular game. Otherwise, any high-exertion aerobic activity will sustain a balanced brain chemistry.

Begin all exercise with a five- to ten-minute warm-up stretching exercise to prepare the muscles for exertion. After your workout, do five to ten minutes of cool-down stretching or walking.

Here's your schedule:

Sunday: Rest and satiation activities.

Monday: Aerobic, arousing exercise activity.

Tuesday: Rest and satiation.

Wednesday: Aerobic, arousing exercise.

Thursday: Rest and satiation.

Friday: Aerobic and arousing exercise.

Saturday: Rest and satiation.

DAILY SCHEDULE

	SUN	MON	TUE	WED	THUR	FRI	SAT
ROUTINE	S	A	S	A	S	A	S

Like food, exercise can be a powerful tool to regulate brain chemistry while it boosts overall health. Most of us think that exercise has no value unless we drive ourselves relentlessly. But science is proving that such beliefs are not only false, but dangerous. When it comes to getting the most out of exercise, the rule of thumb is that moderation is best—a little goes a long way.

In the next chapter, we'll leave the four types of personalities we have been discussing and refine Arousal and Satiation personalities even further, into nine types. When you discover which of the nine types you are, you can tailor your diet, exercise, and lifestyle plans specifically for you.

9

The Nine Personalities

What Type Are You?

A s we've seen, understanding the two general neurochemical types—Arousal and Satiation—is a remarkably effective way to understand the effects of food
and behavior on the brain. But having done more than ten thousand
neurochemical evaluations over the past twenty years, I have found
that greater specificity is not only possible but very useful. For example, you may be an Arousal personality with relatively low norepinephrine, a personality I call the Awakening Warrior; or you may be
an Arousal personality with low serotonin and high dopamine, a type I
call the Armored Knight. Both are Arousal types, yet each is significantly different.

Chapters 10 through 18 will describe the nine personality types
that I've found in my work. Most of us fall into one of these nine types.

Of course, many layers of refinement can be made of these nine, too. Like the Satiation and Arousal personalities, these nine types are generalizations, but they should help you better understand your neurochemical profile—why you are the way you are.

The descriptions of the nine personalities include many characteristics designed to help you better identify and heal your emotional, psychological, and spiritual issues using the brain chemistry model. However, you should not get so attached to the character analysis that you feel restricted or limited in any way. My intention is to help you create a lifestyle that is both healthy and fulfilling. Use whatever information is helpful to you and leave the rest.

As you will see, I draw no clear line separating genetic inheritance, environmental influences, and neurochemistry. Our genes provide us with certain potentials; our environment shapes those potentials. And the two combine to shape the way chemicals act inside the central nervous system.

This section requires a degree of self-reflection and objectivity that may not be easy. It also requires a high degree of participation on your part.

How to Determine Your Neurochemical Personality

The nine personality types are as follows: the Observer, the Awakening Warrior, the Reluctant Runner, the Boatman, the Fretter, the Armored Knight, the Saint, the Fire Starter, and the Mediator. We'll begin with a questionnaire that will help you determine which of these most closely resembles you.

Answer each question with a "yes" or "no," and then add up the total number of "yes" answers from each type. The type with the most "yes" answers is your personality. Once you determine which of the nine personalities is closest to your own, you can read about that personality and the best approach to optimizing your brain chemistry.

Determining Your Neurochemical Personality

Type I: The Observer

1. I am a Satiation person.
2. I prefer quieting and mellowing activities.
3. I am low in serotonin.
4. I like details.
5. I am a very loyal person, sometimes to my detriment.
6. I come from a depressed or compulsive family.
7. I enjoy discussing ideas in small groups.
8. I get anxious rather easily.
9. I am almost "comfortable" with a small amount of depression.
10. I enjoy relationships more than accomplishments.

Type II: The Awakening Warrior

1. I am an Arousal person.
2. I prefer quieting and mellowing activities.
3. I am a serotonin-depleted person.
4. I don't seem to have a lot of rewards in life.
5. I find respect in intelligence and accomplishments.
6. I feel depressed and anxious fairly frequently.
7. I don't meet up to my expectations.
8. I don't need all the details before I get going on a project.
9. I like to make decisions, but am somewhat afraid of failure.
10. I tend to make goals, then don't follow through.

Type III: The Reluctant Runner

1. I am a Satiation person.
2. I prefer exciting and energy-producing activities.

3. I am a serotonin-depleted person.

4. I feel that what I believe I should do is different from what I do.

5. Sometimes I struggle with low energy or depression.

6. I tend to seek the approval of others.

7. I struggle with admitting anything is wrong with me.

8. I find that I offend others very often when I try to offer an opinion.

9. I like to come up with ideas.

10. I struggle with following through on projects, once the excitement is over.

Type IV: The Boatman

1. I am an Arousal person.

2. I prefer exciting and energy-producing activities.

3. I am a serotonin-depleted person.

4. I believe I have been depressed all of my life.

5. When I exercise, I feel good, but for only a short time afterward.

6. I like to learn more about myself and what I need to do to feel better.

7. I believe that I can feel better if I can only find the "key."

8. I am good with people.

9. I tend to encourage others who are feeling bad, even when I feel bad.

10. I am good at following through on a project.

Type V: The Fretter

1. I am a Satiation person.

2. I prefer quieting and mellowing activities.

3. I am a high dopamine person.

4. I am anxious most of the time.

5. My family background is one of anxiety.

6. I often have trouble getting to sleep.

7. I tend to want to control people and situations around me.

8. I like to work on one thing at a time.

9. When I make a change, I need to know why and when it will be over.

10. I don't like it when other people around me are arguing.

Type VI: The Armored Knight

1. I am an Arousal person.

2. I prefer quieting and mellowing activities.

3. I am a high-dopamine person.

4. I am driven to be successful.

5. I feel I need to slow down, but when I do I find it uncomfortable.

6. I am driven more from within than from others.

7. I find myself to be anxious.

8. I find myself liked by almost everyone.

9. I go with the flow, but am also fairly opinionated.

10. I like to stay active.

Type VII: The Saint

1. I am a Satiation person.

2. I prefer exciting and energy-producing activities.

3. I am a high-dopamine person.

4. I get stressed out and feel terrible fairly frequently.

5. I tend to get anxious often.

6. I would love to slow down, but can't.

7. I tend to be a workaholic.

8. I'm good at motivating others.

9. I am creative.

10. I find I have to be careful in relationships not to get too busy for them.

Type VIII: The Fire Starter

1. I am an Arousal person.
2. I prefer exciting and energy producing activities.
3. I am a high-dopamine person.
4. I have lots of energy.
5. I can get bored rather easily and quickly.
6. I am great at getting things going.
7. I struggle with following through with anything to the end.
8. I tend to get sidetracked rather easily.
9. I am a good idea person.
10. I love to work on many projects at the same time.

Type IX: The Mediator

1. I am an Arousal person sometimes and a Satiation person at other times.
2. I don't have a preference for exciting or quieting activities over the other.
3. I don't know if I am high dopamine or low serotonin. It seems I am in the middle.
4. I don't struggle with anxiety any more than I do with depression.
5. I am comfortable with many projects or activities if I am working with people and we are enjoying it.
6. I feel I understand people's problems very well.
7. I like direction, but don't want to be burdened with a lot of detail.
8. I am good at following through with a project.
9. I am comfortable in social situations that include more than one person.
10. I respect people who have balanced their work and family life.

Now count up your "yes" answers for each type. The type that received the most "yeses" is probably yours. Read the chapter about that personality and see how it feels. Now go ahead and read the other chapters too, to determine if one or another better describes you. Don't be tied to your score. If you feel that another personality type is closer to your own, follow the program for that type.

Self-discovery is a world of endless experimentation. It should be both challenging and fun. None of the programs described here is so rigid or so detailed that you cannot shape it to your own needs. The purpose of these chapters is to give you a clearer insight into yourself and start you on the path of using food, exercise, and other behaviors to improve the quality of your life and enhance your performance.

The following nine personalities are extreme examples of types that exist in society. Most of us do not fully embody any one of these nine types. Rather, we resemble one of the nine more than we do any of the others. I have deliberately exaggerated the nine personalities so that people can readily identify each of them, and perhaps better relate to the general characteristics. Most people are much more balanced than these extreme examples. The important thing is to recognize tendencies in yourself and then to see similarities in one or another of the nine personalities. Once you identify the type of personality that best describes your imbalance, you can follow the advice provided to balance your brain chemistry.

That is my goal. I am not at all interested in categorizing people, but in providing clear and accurate guidance to help people achieve healthy neurochemistry. Once that is done, your true—and unique!—nature can emerge.

Finally, you can obtain a more precise analysis of your individual neurochemical profile—and any imbalances that may be present—by filling out the Performance Enhancement Survey provided in the back of this book and sending it in to the Robertson Institute.

10

Type One

The Observer

The Observer is a Satiation type who is genetically predisposed to low serotonin, low dopamine, and low norepinephrine. Though several or all of the major neurotransmitters may be depressed, low serotonin most characterizes the Observer's internal state and outward appearance. In addition, many—though not all—Observers suffer from chronically low energy and often suffer a lack of willpower and self-discipline. They cling to routines and do not like change.

Personality Traits

Like all people, Observers are made up of their own unique balance of strengths and weaknesses, many of which can be understood in terms of their neurochemical profile of low serotonin and/or low dopamine-norepinephrine.

The Observer type comes from a family of people who suffered from low energy and were often emotionally low. Many come from Satiation-type families with depressed or compulsive members who are more comfortable with depression than with arousal. They regard depression as normal, even safe. They dislike stress and avoid excitement. They have a low threshold for arousal and its related elevations of dopamine and norepinephrine. Consequently, the Observer often feels anxious, tense, and insecure. The Observer can suffer from panic attacks whenever dopamine and norepinephrine get too high.

Observers like quieting and inhibiting behaviors, which raise serotonin temporarily. They read, listen to music, watch television, and sometimes stroll in the park—all effective ways of raising serotonin for short periods and creating a sense of safety.

Observers tend to be sedentary people, which relaxes them and raises serotonin somewhat. They assiduously avoid excitement, physically demanding conditions, and adventure, all of which elevate dopamine and norepinephrine. They work unconsciously to keep neurochemistry depressed. This, of course, restricts the kinds of activities Observers allow themselves to participate in, and consequently causes many Observers to feel trapped. Observers who secretly dream of getting out of their rut or improving their circumstances often feel frustrated because they resist the very activities that would make such ambitions possible. Many, however, are happily resigned to their lifestyles, with little ambition of moving beyond their comfortable routines.

For those who do want to change their circumstances, however, depression can be an ongoing problem. They feel victimized and frequently blame others. They don't want to take responsibility for their situation. In the end, that anger tends to melt into self-pity. Observers often eat whenever they are stressed, and because they tend to be sedentary they are often overweight.

In addition to feeling depressed, Observers also suffer from anxiety. The reason is simple: Most people, no matter how hard they try, cannot avoid the standard array of irritations, ups and downs, insecurities, and outright threats to well-being that make up what most people call "normal life." The normal conflicts with co-workers and family members, the insecurities of finances, and the vicissitudes of daily existence all raise dopamine and norepinephrine. Given the fact that Observers are highly sensitive to elevations in the gas-pedal neurotransmitters, they are often chronically anxious, tense, nervous, or downright insecure. As much as possible, they withdraw from intense situations, but they never completely manage to shake off their anxiety and insecurities. These feelings coexist with depression.

Compulsions and Addictions

Such feelings of defeat make the observer vulnerable to an array of compulsions and addictions. Food addictions are the most common, though alcoholism can also affect many. Food is their friend, their comforter, their safety. Observers are often perfectionists when they decide to do something, but paradoxically, they also tend to be procrastinators.

Relationships

Observers can very easily be hurt. They need friendships outside the home to turn to when family matters become intense. They also need time to be alone, quiet, and self-reflective. This allows the Observer to feel safe, to restore his or her sense of boundaries, and to detach from the demands of the external world.

For observers, relationships are often predicated upon an agreement not to reveal the patterns that keep Observers in their ruts. They avoid people who would confront them with the facts of their dilemma and the details of their self-defeating behaviors. This, of course, requires a degree of mutual silence and codependency. For Observers, relationships can also become addictive. They need people; and once they become attached to someone, they form lasting bonds that are very hard for them to break. Because of their insecurities and their repulsion to elevations in dopamine, Observers often struggle to control people and events in their environment in an attempt to maintain safety and low neurochemistry.

Spirituality

Observers approach spiritual life from an emotional and introverted perspective. They are looking for peace, quiet, love, and support. They derive tremendous support from reading spiritual literature, but shy away from big church gatherings, loud singing, and a lot of intense preaching. Those forms of worship are highly arousing and therefore become too stressful. The more Observers understand God as a source of unconditional love and forgiveness, the less stressed, more self-forgiving, and less compulsive they will be. Because Observers are looking for emotional support, they tend to gravitate to emotionally based forms of information rather than intellectual or logical arguments.

The Transformation of the Observer

Observers tend to be incredibly loyal. They love to work for or with strong leaders, people with will, vitality, and vision. It is in these types of relationships that their best abilities emerge. They are good long-range planners.

Observers are wonderful with details. They will stick to a project until it is done perfectly. They have great concentration and can submerge themselves in their work. These qualities make them excellent assistants and secretaries, but they also can become CEOs of their own companies.

Observers are usually highly intelligent and insightful. If they are not running their own business, their loyalty and appreciation for all that the leader or organization provides them—especially the security—combine with their innate talents to bring out the fierce determination to do the best job they can. They are inspired by a strong leader and the struggles he or she may be taking on. They vicariously participate in those struggles, the victories and the defeats. Observers experience the trials and tribulations of life through someone they admire. That is, they experience life at a safe distance. Nevertheless, they will devote themselves entirely to the leader's cause or company, working long hours and doing their best work.

Observers work well in small groups. They want to get along. They want very much to be respected. If they are not respected, or their loyalty is abused, they will turn against the person or organization and become critical, cynical, and a negative force within a company.

Observers need a cause, a company, or a leader to believe in. Though they do not realize it, Observers transform themselves under these conditions. When they are able to dedicate themselves in this way, they are able to push themselves and in the process strengthen their capacity to tolerate dopamine and norepinephrine. Observers will actually engage in the very behaviors they would otherwise resist if they were thinking only of their own lives and their own comforts. They will go to far greater lengths for some*one* or some*thing* than they would have gone to for themselves. Their loyalty triumphs over their fears, and in the process they become happy, highly productive, and incredibly valuable members of a workplace community.

All of these conditions strengthen their neurochemistry. They get psychological rewards for their good work, which pumps up their serotonin levels and their self-esteem. Meanwhile, their hard work promotes the production of dopamine and norepinephrine, which gives them greater will and vitality, and a wider capacity to take on more of the difficulties life presents. As a result, they feel more powerful, more self-motivated, more alive. Depression recedes. Feelings of hope, of expectation, of inner drive emerge. Observers take on bigger tasks—"It must be done for the chief"—and push themselves to accomplish more. In the process, they change their brain chemistry and transform their lives.

The Observer's Program for Peak Performance

If you are an Observer, the bar graph below summarizes the areas that will provide the greatest opportunities for change. The higher the number on the bar graph, the greater the impact of that technique on your brain chemistry.

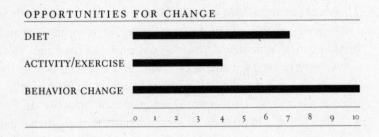

OPPORTUNITIES FOR CHANGE

DIET

ACTIVITY/EXERCISE

BEHAVIOR CHANGE

0 1 2 3 4 5 6 7 8 9 10

Diet

You should eat a diet that is made up primarily of complex carbohydrates, such as whole grains, flour products, vegetables, and fruit. You should also eat low-fat animal products, such as fish, low-fat poultry, and occasionally some skim milk, if desired. The diet for Satiation personality 1 provides the general dietary framework.

This diet will raise serotonin levels and slightly increase dopamine and norepinephrine. You can regulate your dopamine and norepinephrine levels by raising and lowering your protein intake. Follow the dietary suggestions made below and experiment with the frequency with which you eat protein. Monitor yourself to see if your protein consumption is increasing your anxiety. If so, turn more to complex carbohydrates for your staple nutrition.

The diet described below will naturally lower your weight without forcing you to go hungry or even to under-eat. A diet made up primarily of whole grains and low-fat animal foods will lower the fat content of the diet, lower your blood cholesterol, and reduce your weight. It will increase oxygen to your brain and give you plenty of energy. However, if you still feel sluggish, eat more protein foods.

Eat the following foods daily:

- Whole grains: brown rice, barley, millet, oats.
- Flour products: noodles, whole-grain breads, bagels.
- Vegetables for brain chemistry: yams and sweet potatoes, squashes, roots.
- Vegetables for health: green, yellow, orange, and leafy vegetables.

Eat these foods regularly:

- Beans and bean products (tofu): Small amounts, three times per week.
- Fish: Two times per week or more, as long as anxiety and nervous tension do not surface. Lower animal food consumption if anxiety becomes intense or problematical.
- Poultry: Once or twice a week, if desired (preferably without skin). If anxiety increases, eliminate poultry or fish or both until symptoms subside.
- Low-fat dairy products: If desired.

Consider having a complex carbohydrate snack two hours after your protein meal. Possibilities include grain products, such as breads, crackers, muffins, rolls, corn, and chips.

Activity/Exercise

- Serotonin-boosting aerobic exercise will benefit you greatly.
- Walk daily.
- Join a hiking club. Stroll with a partner or a friend.
- Take a low-impact aerobics class.
- Do stretching exercises.

Behavior Change

Behavioral change will bring you the biggest rewards. Among the most important change you can make is to join a small social group or club whose activities are something you genuinely enjoy. Possibilities include book and social clubs; creative writing clubs and workshops; men's and women's groups; small support groups; activities that involve meeting people and developing close friendships. Ideally, the membership in these groups should be small—three, four, or five people. That way, your chances for allowing your innate abilities and talents to shine will be much better. It's vitally important that you are listened to and respected within groups.

Developing close friendships with your spouse and friends is important for you. You need to belong and have acceptance, but must be careful not to discuss problems with others to the point that you stop your need to change. You will need to work on communication techniques to express your opinions without feeling rejected or becoming too aggressive. You can become easily offended and will respond well to talking over your problems with a fellow employee, supervisor, friend, or spouse. You must be careful not to be negative and see only the down side of issues.

When you are under stress, do the following:

- Exercise by walking, stretching, taking a yoga class.
- Eat foods that are rich in complex carbohydrates, such as grains, flour products, and natural sweeteners.
- Avoid highly refined foods, rich in white sugar and artificial ingredients.
- Meditate or pray.
- Involve yourself in family activities, such as with your spouse or children.
- Get out of the house.

- Be among people.
- Share your problems with your spouse or close friend or small support group.

Observers who follow the program can undergo a remarkable change. They are naturally well liked and wonderful team players. Once their inner emotional and psychological condition stabilizes, they have the tools to be successful, effective, and happy.

11

Type Two

The Awakening Warrior

The Awakening Warrior is an Arousal personality who is faced with low serotonin and low norepinephrine, and is consequently biochemically depressed and lacking in energy and will. Specifically, this type must increase norepinephrine and feel comfortable with those increases.

This may sound surprising since this is an Arousal personality, but at the bottom of the Awakening Warrior's personality is a paradox: These are people who are constitutionally active, ambitious, and aggressive, but some type of conditioning—originating either in the nuclear family or through substance abuse in youth—has lowered norepinephrine below its original baseline. Not only is the norepinephrine now lower, but Awakening Warriors have grown used to these lower levels. When norepinephrine rises, they become stressed, anxious, and fearful. In response, they turn to satiation activities in order to drive up serotonin levels and feel safe, but ironically they get little or no reward from satiation.

Deep inside, they see themselves as active, productive, and ambitious. They feel they belong in the struggle of life, but have trouble tolerating it because of all the anxiety it causes. Thus satiating activities make them feel bad about themselves. This contributes physiologically to their depression, though Warriors often do not recognize that they are depressed.

Interestingly, Awakening Warriors do not tend to compensate for their low neurochemistry, except to indulge in satiation behaviors in an attempt to drive up serotonin. The low norepinephrine drives them toward the satiation activities (they shy away from arousal activities). Unfortunately, they don't get much reward from satiation alone—Awakening Warriors need to satisfy both low serotonin and low norepinephrine, but only address the low serotonin imbalance. Since a major part of the personality is left unaddressed, they have a hard time feeling satisfied.

If you are an Awakening Warrior, the warrior within must come into greater prominence within your personality; you must shake your inner warrior out of somnolence in order to change your baseline neurochemistry and begin to enjoy life.

Personality Traits

Awakening Warriors would be able to realize their ambitions were it not for their lack of self-confidence, self-esteem, and the inner drive (thanks to the low norepinephrine) to grasp opportunities. Without these qualities, they indulge excessively in self-defeating behaviors that make them miserable. Unlike Observers, Awakening Warriors are highly uncomfortable with depression. They want to free themselves from it, but don't know how.

The brain chemistry of Awakening Warriors is often an adaptation to conditions that prevailed in the nuclear family or through some type of substance abuse that they exposed themselves to in adolescence or young adulthood.

One way such a neurochemical profile emerges is in the child of alcoholic parents who was brought up in an abusive environment. The conditions within the home not only depressed the young child but also broke his or her will. Thus the child became despondent (low serotonin) and felt unable to affect the situation through aggressive action (causing low norepinephrine). With the decline in serotonin and norepinephrine came a parallel decline in self-esteem. These factors combined and persisted over time to create a new baseline that shaped the personality. This neurochemistry is very present in girls who feel that they cannot fight and thus cannot change the prevailing conditions in the home. They retreat into their own defeated world, which lowers both of the neurotransmitters in question.

This neurochemical profile also emerges in the case of a heavy-handed father who continually berates his son for failing to meet the father's expectations. The son can't do anything right, despite his endless efforts. In time, the son develops a negative and very destructive inner dialogue that reinforces his belief that he is worthless. His inner voice is always saying, "I should have done this," or "I should have done that." He continually negates all the good that he may be doing; but at the same time, the Awakening Warrior knows he can achieve. The problem is that the minute he begins to hope, that negative voice enters his head and consumes him with fear of failure. Thus he has trouble committing to any single direction or work, which of course only confirms his negative inner dialogue. In a sense, Awakening Warriors sabotage themselves.

Arousal personalities may also become Awakening Warriors through a combination of the family scenarios described above and the abuse of drugs or alcohol in adolescence or young adulthood. Many Awakening Warriors feel defeated by their circumstances—they can't relax and feel good, nor do they feel capable of fighting and succeeding. Thus some turn to drugs and alcohol as a way to escape their dilemma. If they use alcohol or marijuana, the drugs may cause them to feel better temporarily, but will also make them increasingly uncomfortable with stressful situations that require effort, will, and struggle. Hence they will retreat even further from life. When they decide that drugs no longer serve them, they will have lost a great deal of confidence and the ability to withstand the pressures of work and ambitious undertakings.

Ironically, once Awakening Warriors reach adulthood or swear off drugs, they generally remain free of addictions. When the passions of adolescence and young adulthood have cooled, they usually do not fall prey to addictive behaviors. They may indulge occasionally in food and may drink alcohol, but not to extremes. In general, Awakening Warriors use quieting activities to raise serotonin, but also suffer from anxiety and nervous tension, the result of elevating norepinephrine levels, with which they are uncomfortable.

Relationships

Awakening Warriors need to develop rewards from relationships, which may be difficult if not approached correctly. Awakening Warriors are in something of a paradox. They are Arousal types, so they're not entirely satisfied with long talks, soft music, and moonlight walks. On the other hand, the low norepinephrine makes it difficult for them to orient their relationships toward activities. But this is precisely what they must do: Turn their social situations into activities and events that require a certain amount of action and doing.

The Transformation of the Awakening Warrior

Awakening Warriors need achievement and success in order to develop a positive self-image. And the most likely way that success can come is by taking aggressive action in the direction of their ambitions. This aggressive action will increase dopamine and norepinephrine and cause them to feel temporarily uncomfortable. That discomfort has been the wall from which they retreat and allows their behavior to become inconsistent. Awakening Warriors need goals and a purpose.

At the same time, however, goals place tremendous pressure on Awakening Warriors to succeed. They have very high expectations. They are performance oriented (again, an Arousal trait), but pessimistic about the outcome of their efforts.

If you are an Awakening Warrior, you might bicycle with friends or a partner, ski, take rugged hikes, climb mountains, drive golf balls, play tennis, bowl, swim. Do fun activities with friends, partners, spouse, and family before engaging in that intimate conversation.

Activity will boost your self-esteem, and also makes you more relaxed and open. You feel as if you've accomplished something and now can be more receptive and flexible with intimate relationships. The combination of activity (Arousal) and intimacy (Satiation) will provide much greater rewards and help you escape the all-too-common trap, which is workaholism and long hours or drudgery at the office.

Awakening Warriors need activity and close relationships, but must understand how to balance their life sufficiently in order to enjoy both. They must first learn how to boost both ends of the neurochemical spectrum in order to enjoy their basic nature, and thus experience the closeness and peace that they are looking for.

Awakening Warriors feel a need to stay busy. They easily become bored and depressed. Also, as social demands increase, anxiety builds. As with relationships, social situations are best when they are based in some type of activity rather than in intimate gatherings or personal discussions. Awakening Warriors prefer to be stimulated from intellectual discussions rather than emotional or personal ones. They feel most comfortable when social activities occur around structured events.

Spirituality

Awakening Warriors tend to be intellectually oriented. They more readily accept information that is grounded in logic or facts than information based on emotion. They approach spiritual matters from an intellectual perspective, and don't really understand the emotional aspect of religion. Faith and surrender are particularly difficult for Awakening Warriors. Religious beliefs are best pursued through the study of theology, by reading spiritual literature, or among other intellectually oriented people involved in small study groups. Without an intellectual basis for religion, Awakening Warriors tend to avoid it, and many such people become very materially oriented.

The Awakening Warrior's Program for Peak Performance

If you are an Awakening Warrior, the bar graph below provides a summary of the methods that will work best for you. The higher the number on the bar graph, the greater the impact that technique will have on your brain chemistry. Behavior change, exercise, and diet will all have profound and positive effects on your brain chemistry, and thus will help alleviate your underlying depression and anxiety. Here is an explanation of all of these techniques.

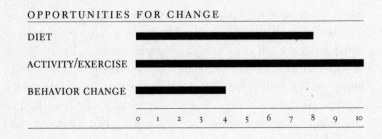

OPPORTUNITIES FOR CHANGE

DIET		
ACTIVITY/EXERCISE		
BEHAVIOR CHANGE		

0 1 2 3 4 5 6 7 8 9 10

Behavior Change

If you are an Awakening Warrior, you must do exactly what the title suggests: Awaken to the warrior within you, which means be consistent in your actions every day and stay with the discomfort that elevations in norepinephrine and dopamine will bring. Specifically, those discomforts are anxiety, insecurity, and tension. These feelings must not put you off your goals. Consistent behavior is a must because only through consistency can your baseline neurochemistry change.

Activity/Exercise

Activity and exercise therapy is essential for emotional and physical health. Activities that provide a measurable way to assess your fitness and progress are particularly rewarding. They build self-esteem and confidence and are essential to your long-term health and brain chemistry balance.

Competitive sports are ideal for you, as long as you do not pin your self-esteem entirely on the outcome of a particular game. You've got to enjoy the game and emphasize competition with yourself; work at improving your skills and use skill development as your central yardstick for progress, as opposed to winning or losing matches. All sports can be played against oneself, as opposed to emphasizing the game against one's opponent, but sports that lend themselves to the "inner game" include skiing, golf, jogging, bicycling, tennis, and many others.

Here are some guidelines for exercise:

1. Try exercising in the morning, before work. This will boost confidence, relax you, and make you feel fit before you take on the challenges of your workday. It will also boost brain chemistry. At first, a good workout will use up dopamine and raise serotonin, but later it will increase dopamine and norepinephrine. An early-morning workout will also increase feelings of well-being and safety before work.

2. Avoid competitive sports when you are feeling particularly anxious, nervous, stressed, or afraid. Instead, do exercises that allow you time to be alone for self-reflection and inner peace. Jog, work out with weights, stretch, do low-impact aerobics, or do some calisthenics on your own.

3. Engage in competitive sports when you are looking for social encounters or want to develop friendships, or feel sufficiently balanced to turn inward and measure your skill development.

Diet

You will respond quickly and powerfully to a healthful diet. You need serotonin and norepinephrine boosters. Use the meal program for Arousal personality 2, along with the following guidelines:

1. When you are feeling weak or suffer from self-doubt, eat a high-protein meal and avoid carbohydrates. Use protein to boost inner strength and outer strength.

2. When you are feeling stressed and anxious, eat a high-carbohydrate meal and avoid protein. Use carbohydrate to lower tension, anxiety, and stress, and to gain inner peace.

3. Avoid refined white sugar at all times. It will temporarily elevate serotonin but negatively affect blood sugar and moods by lowering blood sugar shortly after consumption.

4. Eat a high-protein meal at least once a day.

5. Make your protein meals low fat, such as fish or the white meat of poultry.

6. Experiment with protein in the morning.

Diet can be very beneficial for your brain. You should start to see results from your diet in a week or two.

As an Awakening Warrior, you are stronger than you think. That is the source of your psychological and neurochemical problems. Your transformation comes when you commit to using your strength and enduring the temporary discomfort that competitive activities bring. When you see yourself in more heroic terms, and act on that heroic self-image, there is nothing that can stop you—you already have the talent and the power to become the very person you secretly believe yourself to be.

12

Type Three

The Reluctant Runner

The Reluctant Runner is one of the most prevalent neurochemical profiles in America today. It is particularly common among young to middle-aged people who are engaged in business, the media, and the law. Constitutionally, Reluctant Runners are Satiation personalities, but they push themselves into workaholism—in part because of their own ambitions, but especially because they find themselves in environments in which they are rewarded for being aggressive, hardworking, dedicated to the job, and constantly driving themselves beyond their limits. In other words, norepinephrine and dopamine rule the day.

Specifically, the brain chemistry profile of Reluctant Runners is low serotonin and low norepinephrine; but unlike Awakening Warriors, they are Satiation types. Also unlike Awakening Warriors, Reluctant Runners compensate effectively for low norepinephrine, but neglect the serotonin. The Runners are usually good athletes. They like exercise and competition. They were also good students and are naturally smart.

Personality Traits

I call them Reluctant Runners because in their heart of hearts, they are family-centered lovers who really want to develop close, intimate relationships but are pushed to work hard and succeed by the prevailing pressures of cultural expectation, the demands of employers, financial pressures, and personal ambition. Runners are continually pushing themselves to work harder, give more to their jobs, and refrain from asking for more time to be with their families. This internalized voice drives them to feel insecure about their jobs and their professional futures.

Interestingly, Reluctant Runners are almost always good at their jobs. They seek approval from their employers and colleagues, and they want the benefits of success. What they don't want to think about are the costs. Whenever that subject comes up, even unprovoked within themselves, they push it aside. Many so-called "yuppies" are Reluctant Runners.

Reluctant Runners suffer a personal and spiritual conflict because, on one hand, they possess humanistic and spiritual ideals that cause them to yearn for a balanced life. Yet the Runners somehow neglect those values and even live in opposition to them. Eventually, the contradiction leads to a personal crisis. Until that point, many Runners push themselves to achieve professionally, working late at night and weekends. Meanwhile, they suffer pangs of the heart whenever their children ask them to play and they have to say no because there's too much work to be done. They are moving too fast for their own good, and eventually something within the psyche rears up and says, "It's time to stop what you're doing and start smelling the linseed oil in your child's baseball glove."

Thus Reluctant Runners reach the age of forty or forty-five and suffer the inevitable midlife crisis, with all its questioning and soul searching. The neglect of the serotonin side of the personality, the neglect of all those wonderful Satiation activities, has created an imbalance that leads to a need to realign and redirect one's life.

In order to stifle the demands of the Satiation personality, Runners self-medicate by drinking coffee, eating high-protein foods, working hard, and exercising—all of which will boost dopamine and norepinephrine levels. Beneath the high-anxiety lifestyle that Runners lead is depression, which they deny and push away by revving up the stress level and becoming preoccupied with their fear of slipping on the career ladder or simply losing their job. Like low serotonin, low norepinephrine also leads to depression, but Runners manage to keep up their norepinephrine levels by virtue of their lifestyle. Thus when Runners wake up feeling low, they drink coffee, go to the gym, race around doing errands, and push themselves hard at work.

Relationships

As Satiation personalities, Runners prefer intimacy and close relationships. They seek approval from others, but especially within the professional world. Indeed, very often they put more stock in what others think than in what they themselves think. This, of course, plays right into their need to push themselves harder, especially for those at work. Also, it makes them very vulnerable to being emotionally hurt. Nevertheless, their major rewards will come from relationships, rather than achievements and activity.

Reluctant Runners are emotional and heart-centered. They tend to accept information that is emotionally based rather than strictly intellectual and logical.

Like all people, Runners need people they can trust; but unlike many, they are capable of trust and intimacy. They are better in small groups in which personal and emotional issues can be discussed and people can open up to one another. It's very important for Runners to feel respected; but once they are assured of respect, they can let down their guard and develop strong friendships.

Reluctant Runners are less fond of socializing with large groups. Indeed, parties play right into their low-norepinephrine issues: They have trouble relaxing; they push themselves to be witty and showy; and they get very caught up with their own personas. All of these kinds of social responses will drive up norepinephrine. Yet the whole experience leaves them feeling exhausted and wondering why they bother.

Compulsions and Addictions

Because a powerful inner conflict underlies the Runner personality, they often suffer addictions and compulsions. Runners become perfectionists and control oriented and suffer from binge eating at times. They also procrastinate, a function of their Satiation reward center. Reluctant Runners tend to drink alcohol, but not necessarily to excess. They need the approval of others—especially in their work—which makes it unlikely that they will become alcoholics. If they become addicted to alcohol, it is usually after their midlife crisis—not before. On the other hand, Runners can become addicted to drugs, either marijuana to help them relax or cocaine to help them perform. Many Reluctant Runners are the baby boomers who are driving themselves to make it in the material world, yet have strong spiritual values beneath the surface. This conflict makes it difficult for them to give themselves entirely to material success. When the pressure to perform becomes great enough, however, they can easily succumb to drugs that promote the gas-pedal neurotransmitters. Cocaine is the most likely choice.

Spirituality

Though spiritual values are very important to the Runners, they are often given to New Age thinking and may not be members of a specific religion. Whatever religion they participate in, however, they will take an emotional perspective toward their faith and spiritual views. Forgiveness, unconditional love, and acceptance are central themes in their vocabulary, but they do not believe them sufficiently to risk surrendering to God. Hence they remain control oriented, seemingly self-sufficient, and secretly afraid of what lies around the corner.

Transformation of the Reluctant Runner

Reluctant Runners look great from the outside. All this dedication to work usually gives them some measure of material success. They tend to be athletic and youthful looking, and often seem to have it all — until the game breaks open and they get divorced, lose their jobs, suffer a financial crisis, or contract some type of illness. Then the whole pretense unravels and they begin to look deeply at their lives.

For Reluctant Runners, a midlife crisis very often brings rebirth and renewal. Somehow, the caterpillar becomes the butterfly. The trick is for them to reorient toward their underlying Satiation reward center. If they continue to push and struggle with their will, they often suffer the proverbial crash. But if they reflect on their lives and reconnect with the true underlying values, they undergo a new integration in which the inner beliefs and the outer lifestyle come into greater harmony. Runners are often the people who you hear saying, "I used to be one of those clones up there in that office, until my wife walked out on me and my daughter got sick. Then I stopped seeing the world only through the rearview mirror of my BMW." Remarkably, Reluctant Runners often find the way toward a better existence after the fall. They emerge for the better, in large measure because they are true to their reward center.

The Reluctant Runner's Program for Peak Performance

If you are a Reluctant Runner, your health depends on restoring balance in your life. The bar graph on the next page summarizes the kinds of techniques you can use to restore neurochemical balance to your life. The higher the number on the bar graph, the greater the impact that technique will have on your brain chemistry.

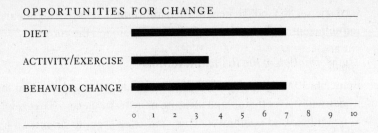

Behavior Change

For Reluctant Runners, behavioral change, exercise, and diet will have profound effects on brain chemistry, as the bar graph demonstrates. Behavioral change means literally spending more time in satiation activities. The first and most important is for you to be truly present and awake to the love of your spouse, children, and other important people in your life. Slow down, taking more time to self-reflect. Engage in artistic pursuits, such as painting, sculpting, or writing. Take up a hobby that you enjoy and want to get better at. Learn something that you always dreamed of studying but never got around to. Spend time in pursuits that enrich you but will have no apparent impact on your income or career. Review your spiritual beliefs. Go to church or synagogue. Talk to people with open minds and strong spiritual beliefs. Develop the more passive, gentle, and receptive parts of your being. All of these activities will give you tremendous rewards by significantly boosting serotonin levels and making you feel more whole.

Activity/Exercise

You may be involved in some type of exercise program already, or you may have trouble following a specific exercise regimen. You must choose something you enjoy doing and it must be coupled with satiation activities. Choose one of the satiation exercise programs described in chapter 8. Walking daily is especially important to work off stress and restore a positive self-image. Competitive games are wonderful for Runners, but they must be joined with satiation activities if you are committed to attaining balance. Balance your tennis or basketball game, for example, with walking or stretching.

Diet

Diet can have a profound effect on neurochemistry, and will likely have an impact that you can feel and understand within a few weeks. Use the following guidelines to help you with choosing foods:

1. Use a modified version of the food program for Satiation personality 1 described in chapter 7.

2. Make complex carbohydrates, such as whole grains, whole-grain breads, pastas, bagels, and flour products your central foods.

3. Eat lots of vegetables (especially potatoes, squash, and roots) and fruit.

4. For protein foods, eat fish, the white meat of poultry, and low-fat dairy products (if you desire them).

5. Avoid red meat and eggs.

6. Try to limit high-protein foods to once a day or three times a week.

7. Eat high-protein foods when you need a boost in self-confidence or personal power or when preparing for a special meeting or presentation.

8. Eat whole grains, flour products, and sweets to help you relax.

9. Avoid white sugar to prevent wide swings in blood sugar.

10. Avoid the following foods or eat them sparingly: pickled herring; pork and pork products; whole milk; most cheeses, especially cheddar, Stilton, and Camembert (high in protein and fat); ripe bananas (loaded with sugar); raisins; avocados; liver; canned figs.

11. Avoid caffeine or eat sparingly, including coffee, chocolate, and other caffeine-containing products.

12. Avoid or minimize alcohol.

Reluctant Runners know that a spiritual crisis looms unless they redirect their lives toward the things they truly love. It doesn't seem all that difficult to make such a change, except when all your time is consumed by your work and responsibilities—or so it seems. Change is a necessity, and with time and faith, you can slow down and learn to walk.

13

Type Four

The Boatman

T he Boatman has an Arousal reward center, with low serotonin and high dopamine-norepinephrine. This combination can be challenging because the person can be both depressed and anxious. A small percentage of people with this neurochemical profile are a bit manic, and an even smaller group are self-destructive. The vast majority, however, are seekers of truth and understanding.

Personality Traits

Boatmen are growth oriented and eager to try anything to get themselves free of their depression and anxiety. They will pursue any avenue, try any self-improvement program, and engage in any new technique, all in an effort to understand themselves and achieve some degree of balance and harmony within. Unfortunately, all this "doing" often amounts to a self-defeating struggle. The reason is that activity elevates an already high dopamine level and does nothing for the low serotonin.

I call these people Boatmen because for them achieving balance means sailing smoothly along the river of life toward their goals rather than struggling against the stream, as they tend to do. If they would relax and enjoy life a little bit—let the river carry them—they would elevate serotonin almost effortlessly, and lower norepinephrine.

There's a very good reason why Boatmen do not simply ride the waves with ease. Depression and anxiety together are very difficult to tame, especially if you know nothing of the neurochemical model. The two moods pull in different directions. Depression causes most people to retreat. Anxiety causes many to advance and try to directly influence the situation at hand.

When faced with the decision of whether to retreat or advance, Arousal personalities typically decide to tackle the problems head-on. In one way or another, they struggle against their issues. Many go to therapy. Others seek answers from doctors or people who are wise or have some new form of treatment. In short, many Arousal types actively pursue their goals.

Much of this activity is designed to cover up the fact that Boatmen are also biochemically depressed. They struggle to avoid depression by staying busy, which pumps up dopamine and norepinephrine. When these gas-pedal neurotransmitters become too high, however, Boatmen experience anxiety, stress, and restlessness.

One of the reasons they act aggressively is the neurochemical profile itself: Dopamine causes aggression. Another is the fact that our society rewards people for activity and looks critically on those who take a more relaxed approach to life. Thus the neurochemical and social demands combine to push people with this kind of profile toward hard work and struggle, which often makes their life miserable.

In fact, activity—especially high-intensity exercise, which is very common among the Boatman types—provides a short-term reward.

Exercise uses dopamine and norepinephrine and causes a temporary rise in serotonin. But this is a short-term balance. Eventually, dopamine rises to its baseline levels (sometimes even higher) and serotonin falls. In the end, Boatmen often feel let down, distraught, and hopeless. They have done everything right—sought therapy, worked out—yet nothing seems to help. In the end, they have difficulty getting rewards from their compensatory behavior.

First and foremost, Boatmen must realize that their lack of performance is not just psychological, but physiological. In fact, they may have a stronger physiological imbalance than any psychological disturbance. Yet they experience the issues as psychological because they are related to moods—either depression, or anxiety, or both—and pursue the standard psychological answers, which often don't work. Most Boatmen were born with this imbalance. Their neurochemical profile is grounded in their genes. As children, they suffered from low serotonin and depression.

Exercise is particularly paradoxical for Boatmen. They probably go to the gym, work out for thirty minutes or an hour, sweat profusely, and emerge from their exercise regimen feeling really good. Serotonin is up and so are feelings of well-being, self-confidence, and self-esteem. Unfortunately, serotonin soon falls, while dopamine and norepinephrine rise. With the gas-pedal neurotransmitters come anxiety, stress, and depression. Naturally, they believe they've got to spend more time in the gym to cure themselves, but that is only going to make matters worse. Their behavior is sabotaging them, but they don't know it. They feel they're doing everything right, but nothing seems to work for any length of time. With the right program, however, Boatmen can enhance their performance.

Relationships

As with other Arousal types, Boatmen have the easiest time relating to others when they are involved in some type of arousal activity. A Boatman's neurochemical profile will show a preference for action and activities that have a purpose. Satiation activities make them restless, bored, and eventually depressed. Married Boatmen find that arousal activities with their family provide a sense of closeness and relaxation. Family events that include such activities as playing baseball, tennis, or basketball; skiing, fishing, or boating; camping, hiking, or swimming—all of these are ideal. They utilize and lower dopamine and norepinephrine, while they raise serotonin levels.

Compulsions and Addictions

Like other Arousal types, Boatmen must be careful of extremes. On one hand, they can easily become workaholics and shut out their family or loved ones. On the other, they must avoid boredom, which turns into depression.

Boatmen must be careful not to become overly competitive or controlling with others. This indicates an over-reliance on arousal and dopamine, which means they are becoming overly aggressive and bordering on violence.

Spirituality

Boatmen approach spiritual beliefs from an intellectual perspective. Emotional ideals and faith are often difficult to comprehend. They may be comfortable in developing their spiritual lives through study of spiritual literature, within a structured setting. Boatmen tend to accept information that is intellectually based, rather than emotional in nature. If they're not careful, they can succumb to exclusively materialistic goals, which would mean that they are neglecting the satiation side of the personality.

Transformation of the Boatman

Ironically, I have found that faith is part of the answer for Boatmen. They benefit enormously from developing spiritual beliefs and faith that allow them to relax and protect them from all the possibilities that they fear and struggle against. Only through faith can they learn to let go and allow the river of life to carry them forward. Only in this way can Boatmen allow their more receptive side to emerge and thus allow serotonin production to develop.

The Boatman's Program for Peak Performance

If you are a Boatman, you must learn balance. You must learn to satisfy both your satiation and arousal needs. The bar graph below summarizes which techniques will have the greatest impact on your brain chemistry. The higher the number on the bar graph, the greater the impact of that technique.

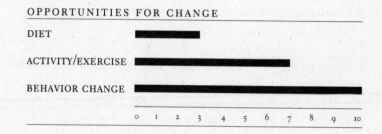

OPPORTUNITIES FOR CHANGE

DIET	
ACTIVITY/EXERCISE	
BEHAVIOR CHANGE	

0 1 2 3 4 5 6 7 8 9 10

Behavior Change

In attempting to achieve balance, you must begin by developing a relationship with at least one other person whom you trust and love; someone with whom, over time, you can learn to share your inner self. You must also find a place that provides you a safe haven where you can relax and shut out the world.

Activity/Exercise

Follow the exercise plan for Arousal personality 2 (described in chapter 8), which is designed for people with low serotonin and high dopamine. You can enjoy competitive sports if you can avoid placing your entire self-worth on the game's outcome. Be careful to check yourself against any overly aggressive behavior, which can emerge under intense competitive conditions.

Follow these guidelines in conjunction with your workout:

1. Before you do any arousal exercises, perform five to ten minutes of warm-up (satiation) exercises, such as walking, stretching, and some gentle calisthenics.
2. Perform at least twenty minutes of rigorous aerobic or weight training from the arousal list (see chapter 8).
3. After you've exercised, perform another round of walking and gentle stretching (satiation).

Whenever you feel stressed or anxious, perform exercises from the arousal list and follow that with some stretching or yoga.

Diet

Diet can be very beneficial for your neurochemical balance. You will want to determine if you begin to "feel better" after a few weeks on the plan. The best diet for you is the one described in the diet for Arousal personality 1, for types with low serotonin (described in chapter 8).

Here are some additional guidelines:

1. Whenever you are feeling weak or lacking in confidence, eat protein foods. This guideline applies especially when you face a particularly demanding work schedule or must given an important presentation.
2. When you are stressed, anxious, and tense, eat carbohydrate foods.
3. Reduce or eliminate refined white sugar to avoid extremes in blood sugar levels, energy, and moods.
4. Avoid red meat, eggs, and high-fat dairy products.
5. Eat fish, poultry, beans, and low-fat dairy products for your protein.

Here's an old trick that all of us learned in childhood: Two children are playing tug-of-war with a rope. They are evenly matched, so they struggle but neither one gains the upper hand. Suddenly, one of them gets the bright idea to let go of the rope, which sends the other child hurtling backward and flat on the ground. At that point, the one who has let go can pull the rope free or drag his helpless opponent across the loser's line.

Boatmen can gain a great deal from this strategy. You shouldn't struggle so much against life—that only results in a standoff, at best. Most of the time, it causes you feelings of frustration and loss. But the minute you relax, you start to win. Learn to let go of the rope once in a while. You'll soon see that when you stop wasting your considerable strength on hopeless struggle and work with the momentum instead of against it, much of life will become considerably easier.

14

Type Five

The Fretter

The Fretter is a Satiation personality with abnormally high dopamine and low serotonin, causing high anxiety. As a result, worry colors the entire background of the person's life. Fretters are continually doing things that they hope will cause relaxation or at least distraction from worry. However, in the Fretter's case, the worry is self-promoting, since such feelings continually drive up dopamine levels and thus promote more intense feelings of insecurity and fear. Fretters see virtually every moment as rife with hidden dangers. Many adults become Fretters later in life.

Personality Traits

Fretters are usually highly compulsive and high-strung. They frequently smoke cigarettes, drink coffee and alcohol, and indulge in an endless array of rituals and perfectionistic behaviors. Eventually, most forms of stimulation become too arousing for Fretters and thus contribute to their worried state. In response, they try to control their environments, often by limiting the size and scope of their worlds. Unless they gain control of their neurochemistry, many Fretters end up in single-room apartments or—if they live in big houses—wall themselves off within one part of the house, which they use as a kind of bunker against the threats they believe are outside the front door.

Fretters come from Fretters, meaning their parents and siblings often suffer from elevated dopamine, too. They are genetic worriers. However, it must be understood that Fretters engage in activities that drive up dopamine and thereby maintain their own condition. High dopamine has become their baseline, so that behaviors that maintain high dopamine are rewarding, in a kind of self-destructive way. Once dopamine gets too high, Fretters look for ways to calm themselves. Unfortunately, those calming behaviors often become compulsions or addictions.

Fretters can alleviate their intense internal issues by engaging in behaviors that lower dopamine and increase serotonin. This will make them worry less and will promote feelings of well-being. Until they take up such measures, however, Fretters will live on a treadmill on which worry begets dopamine, which begets more worry.

Compulsions and Addictions

Fear drives the Fretters' daily lives. Their compulsiveness causes them to rigidly structure their day. They become attached to their schedules because they see them as forms of safety, buttresses against intrusions from the outside world. Fretters don't like people to drop over to their house; they don't like sudden news or requests for get-togethers for which they are unprepared. They are continually trying to smooth out their days, calm the waters of life, and avoid change. They often view disruptions in their schedule as personal attacks. They will argue irrationally with their relatives for the sanctity of their schedules. Their relatives, on the other hand, usually do not understand the need Fretters have for some degree of safety, which their concretized schedules provide. Hence Fretters are often surrounded by conflict, which drives up dopamine further.

Instead of addressing their beliefs and behaviors, Fretters usually look for a quick fix. They turn to medication, cigarettes, television, or alcohol for solace and comfort, all of which can become addictive. Many of the people addicted to tranquilizers and sleeping pills are Fretters. Though these addictions may provide some very temporary relief, they ultimately fail the Fretter and tend to make matters worse. Sleeping pills and many of the milder tranquilizers work by elevating GABA, an inhibitor that induces sleep. Since dopamine isn't lowered by such drugs, it remains a source of anxiety.

In addition to the above-mentioned addictions, Fretters also are given to compulsions involving food, procrastination, and ritual.

Relationships

Fretters prefer close personal friendships and one-on-one interactions. Within a family, Fretters can become overly concerned about the safety and emotional well-being of their children or siblings. Socially, Fretters are at their best when they are in a safe, structured, and comfortable setting. Exciting activities or social events trigger anxiety and stress for Fretters. On the other hand, Fretters love their children and enjoy safe activities and the feeling of being close. Fretters must learn to be clear about what works for them in social situations, especially with the people they want to be close to. If they make clear requests of their spouse and children, they can create more harmonious interactions that Fretters can truly enjoy.

If Fretters have nothing to worry about for themselves, they will worry about their children, or a friend, or the state of the world. They never realize that it is a powerful and negative belief system that causes such worry. All this worry and internal stress often leads to depression.

To balance social demands, Fretters need quiet periods alone, to self-reflect and feel the safety of their own boundaries.

Spirituality

Fretters tend to approach their spiritual lives from an emotional perspective. They need and want to be loved. They need to believe in forgiveness, unconditional love, and reconciliation. Indeed, it is their fear of some horrible thing happening to them that is partially responsible for their elevated dopamine levels. This, in its essence, is a spiritual problem. As Albert Einstein put it, we all must decide if the universe is a friendly place. Beneath all their rationalizations and sugar-coated truths, Fretters clearly answer that question with a "no."

Transformation of the Fretter

Because Fretters perceive the world as dangerous, a strong spiritual life is part of the Fretter's solution. The comfort that comes with faith promotes serotonin production and provides some sense of well-being and safety.

Fretters must understand that they are not alone. Fears of disaster and tragedy always have been central to the human condition, just as faith, spirituality, and religious practices have been humanity's primary buttress against the vicissitudes of life. The fears Fretters experience are calmed, and serotonin levels rise, when Fretters learn to pray and participate in a spiritual community. The right community can offer friendship, support, and a sense of shared struggle, all of which help Fretters avoid the trap of loneliness and isolation that fear can so easily create.

The Fretter's Program for Peak Performance

If you are a Fretter, the bar graph below summarizes the kinds of techniques that will help you lower dopamine and raise serotonin. The higher the number on the bar graph, the greater the impact of that particular technique on your brain chemistry.

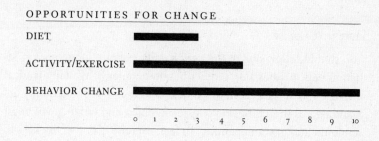

OPPORTUNITIES FOR CHANGE

DIET

ACTIVITY/EXERCISE

BEHAVIOR CHANGE

0 1 2 3 4 5 6 7 8 9 10

Behavior Change

Behavioral change (including exercise and diet) will have the greatest impact on your health and well-being. The first thing that you need — though you are probably loathe to do it — is psychological and spiritual help. The counselor's or clergyman's office is the perfect setting for you. It is a safe place to confront your fears, to see the irrational nature of your anxiety, and to begin to implement different and more constructive behaviors in daily life. You can see either a counselor or a clergyman or both — whatever your preference.

Regardless, you must inculcate some sort of faith system into your life if you are to escape the tyranny of fear and anxiety. The safety of the counselor's or clergy's office alone will increase serotonin and decrease dopamine. Whether counselor or clergy, this helping professional acts as an anchor in your upending sea.

The life-affirming point of view imparted by the counselor is a direct confrontation of your fears. Part of the therapy should be to lead you into your fears and discover what it is that you are so afraid of. This can happen much more easily in a safe setting. When the inner villain has been exposed and acknowledged as a false fear, it can be brought into clearer perspective. Before that can happen, of course, you must agree to seek counseling and then develop trust for your counselor. Ultimately, you must change your view of life and see that there is far more protection and safety than you currently believe.

Activity/Exercise

You should follow one of the gentle daily exercise programs for Satiation personalities 1 or 2, described in chapter 8. Walking is ideal because it is aerobic, it boosts fitness, and it can be increasingly demanding. All stretching, low-impact aerobics, and walking will boost serotonin and lower dopamine. In fact, exercise is one of the keys to your recovery.

Diet

If you are like most Fretters, you probably tend to eat foods that are rich in protein, easy to prepare, and low in nutritional value. Among the most common foods eaten by Fretters are minute steaks, hamburgers, chicken, and eggs. They tend to like prepared meals, such as TV dinners. Their desserts, if they eat any at all, are usually loaded with sugar. Fretters often have poor appetites, so their demands are usually small.

You can help yourself tremendously simply by eating more healthful foods. Follow these guidelines:

1. Follow the diet for Satiation personality 1, low-serotonin types, described in chapter 7.

2. Significantly reduce all protein foods.

3. Significantly reduce or eliminate all red meat (including steaks, hamburgers, and bacon) and eggs.

4. Eat fish, beans, and the white meat of chicken as your source of protein.

5. Rely on complex carbohydrates as the primary source of your nutrition.

6. Eat a complex carbohydrate meal or snack whenever fear, tension, or anxiety become excessive.

7. Avoid all caffeinated foods and beverages—above all, stop drinking coffee.

8. Avoid alcohol.

Once you begin to feel some sense of safety and comfort, your underlying strengths and abilities will come forward, especially your natural capacity to care for and support others. When such caring is combined with a sense of personal safety, your true nature will be revealed: no longer worrying, but loving, supportive, and kind.

15

Type Six

The Armored Knight

The Armored Knight is an Arousal personality with low to normal serotonin and normal to high dopamine who gets rewarded for pushing up the gas-pedal neurotransmitters. Armored Knights have tremendous drive, energy, and the will to achieve their professional goals and are usually highly successful. They have knowledge, intelligence, and power and are often leaders who command respect.

Beneath the surface competence, however, lies an extreme imbalance. Armored Knights have great difficulty slowing down and being present with their close relationships. When dopamine gets too high, they withdraw into their own world or vegetate around the house, barely communicating, as if they have reverted to an opposite personality. Normally extroverted and tremendously energetic, they push themselves hard each day until the dopamine and norepinephrine levels get too high, at which point they finally shut down and withdraw into their armor. Then they are available to no one.

They withdraw because they get no reward from satiation activities that involve other people. Many Armored Knights would love to be able to carry off their professional lives and still be available to spouse, children, or other loved ones. In fact, they secretly long to relax and be good parents. However, intimacy and loving relationships usually require Armored Knights to slow down too much for their brain chemistry to tolerate, which means they become depressed. Physiologically, they must slow down because dopamine has become exceedingly elevated. At that point, they become anxious and tense. They must slow down and allow the gas-pedal neurotransmitters to recede. As dopamine and norepinephrine levels fall, they feel less intense and less aggressive. This would be the perfect time to be close to family or friends. Unfortunately, there's not enough serotonin available at these times to impart a feeling of well-being and safety. This means that there's a background issue of depression and the absence of well-being. Thus when dopamine levels are falling, Armored Knights feel vulnerable and on the edge. Intimacy feels threatening. Instead of wanting to be around others, they seek refuge within their armored exterior.

Personality Traits

Many Armored Knights were raised by parents with Arousal personalities who pushed their children to succeed but avoided intimacy themselves. Their families were constantly on the go. One of the central methods the parents used to push their children was criticism, which created psychological wounds. Armored Knights escaped the pain of those wounds by being busy and by achieving success.

As children, Armored Knights were very creative, highly intelligent, and active. They had innate abilities that would form the foundation for success. Unfortunately, their parents' criticism made the

Armored Knights deeply afraid of failure. Such fear only caused them to work harder and to be more heavily invested in success. Within their family, success wasn't something merely to be admired or appreciated, but was essential to survival. This inordinate need for achievement restricted their natural expressiveness, their joy for learning, playing, and having fun. The pain of the criticism also made intimacy—even intimacy with themselves—difficult, if not impossible.

As adults, Armored Knights still find intimacy dangerous. They would rather vegetate in front of the television set—a safe way to promote serotonin and lower dopamine. It also helps them avoid being with people and facing the demands of family.

Compulsions and Addictions

Armored Knights are prone to workaholism and all activities that drive up dopamine. They arc risk takers and can easily become compulsive gamblers. Like other Arousal personalities, Armored Knights are also vulnerable to cocaine addiction. They also tend to drink alcohol, and some can do it to excess.

For most people, alcohol is a way of dampening dopamine and raising serotonin; therefore it is often used to trigger retreat into oneself. However, since that retreat is short-lived for most Armored Knights, they do not tend to overindulge in alcohol. They're looking for longer-lasting retreats. There are circumstances that can lead Knights to become alcoholics, however. For instance, they are especially vulnerable when thrown into long-term crises at work, crises that are personally threatening and continually elevate dopamine and norepinephrine. At that point, alcohol becomes a form of self-medication to keep dopamine levels down, especially at night, when they want to escape their dopamine-stoked day and start to relax.

Relationships

As with other Arousal personalities, Armored Knights are most comfortable when social situations are structured and tied to some form of activity. They like to *do* things with others more than they like having intimate and personal conversations. Indeed, their conversations tend to center around business or shop talk, rather than on how a friend might feel about personal issues in his or her life. If the conversation turns toward the emotional or aesthetic subjects, Knights become bored and maybe even depressed.

These characteristics are true even when Knights are dealing with family members. Thus Armored Knights are at their best in structured activity. They are better at playing baseball or basketball or tennis with their children than they are at having heart-to-heart talks or exploring emotions.

When activities slow down, anxiety starts to build. Armored Knights tend to allow the anxiety to escalate or attempt to avoid it until it overwhelms them. At that point, they either withdraw or explode with anger to let off steam.

Spirituality

Armored Knights will generally approach their spiritual beliefs from an intellectual perspective. Emotional arguments or discussions of faith are difficult for them to truly comprehend. The study of spiritual literature may hold some interest for them, but many will avoid this as well. Armored Knights tend to be materially oriented, at least until they can slow down and appreciate the need for satiation activities and serotonin.

Armored Knights have no underlying conflict with their values. Instead, they have difficulty being in relationship with their tender, vulnerable, and emotional side. Since spiritual life lies at the core of such feelings, they are cut off from such fundamental spiritual precepts as unconditional love, forgiveness, and reconciliation. Until they open up to this side, they will see spiritual life as essentially foreign.

Transformation of the Armored Knight

Armored Knights must learn to take off their armor. To do that, they must first elevate their serotonin levels. Meanwhile, they've got to become more comfortable with serotonin and satiation activities, neither of which feel particularly good nor particularly rewarding. All the Armored Knights' rewards are tied up with dopamine. Every time they slow down, the child inside feels threatened, under attack by bigger, more powerful people. Hence slowing down and doing anything other than achievement-oriented activities is highly threatening and adds to their anxiety.

Armored Knights are particularly vulnerable to certain types of life crises. Among the most common are divorce (because of their tendency to avoid intimacy and neglect their spouses), illness (because they can abuse their bodies as they drive themselves toward success), and some type of financial collapse. When any of these crises emerge, they have the opportunity to address the more receptive, open, and spiritual sides of themselves. At that point, transformation is not only possible, but likely.

The Armored Knight's Program for Peak Performance

The bar graph below summarizes the effectiveness of the techniques that will be helpful to you in balancing neurochemistry. The higher the number on the bar graph, the greater the impact that technique will have on your brain chemistry.

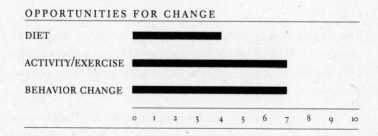

OPPORTUNITIES FOR CHANGE

Behavior Change

The central behavioral change that you need to make is to open up the feeling side of life. You must become more comfortable with your emotions and those of others, especially those in your family. Intimacy with loved ones is the key to your learning to be comfortable with satiation and serotonin. You must recognize that time and life are short and that your spouse, children, and loved ones need your love and appreciation at a deep emotional level. Love and appreciation for family and friends, in fact, are key to your transformation. These people are sufficiently important in your life to get you to slow down and spend time getting to know them. As you do, you will be forced to deal with your own emotional scars and, in the process, your baseline neurochemistry will change toward higher serotonin and slightly lower dopamine. You will very likely always be an Arousal personality, but such elevated dopamine levels are not necessary in order to be effective and successful. A whole side of your being, with all its joys, sadness, and rich rewards, awaits exploration.

Activity/Exercise

The exercise program for Arousal personality 2 (described in chapter 8) is ideal for you. All competitive sports, all aerobic workouts, and games that involve skill development and self-improvement are perfect for you. In addition, regular walks with your family will elevate serotonin and make it easier for you to feel close without feeling inordinately threatened.

Diet

The diet for Arousal personality 1 with low serotonin (described in chapter 7) will be helpful to you, and should have a noticeable effect within a few weeks. Meanwhile, follow these guidelines, especially when you are feeling anxious or depressed:

1. Whenever you feel anxious, stressed, and afraid, reduce or eliminate animal protein and make complex carbohydrates the central part of your diet—at least until the symptoms abate.

2. When you feel that your thoughts are out of focus or scattered, or whenever you must concentrate on a single subject, eat complex

carbohydrates. (See chapters 5 and 8 for more information on special enhancers and optimal diets, respectively.)

3. Reduce or eliminate all red meat, hard cheese, and eggs.

4. Make fish, poultry, beans, and low-fat dairy foods your primary protein foods.

5. Whenever you are faced with a demanding business meeting, eat fish or some other low-fat, high-protein food to optimize brain chemistry and promote increased neurotransmission.

You face a new adventure and challenge, one that lies within. You must see that it is your own dragons that drive you away from the most precious of all gifts in life, the love of family and friends. Only you can slay those dragons. But once you take up the challenge, you are fully capable of succeeding.

16

Type Seven

The Saint

The Saint is a Satiation personality with low serotonin and high dopamine, which means that anxiety and fear is at the center of the Saint's personality. Saints try to control their anxiety by pleasing others, but feel that they are continually falling short and never fully experience satisfaction. Saints have high dopamine and norepinephrine, but get no reward for boosting these gas pedals further. They are anxious to begin with, and as the demands in their lives increase, they get more anxious, stressed, and fearful.

Personality Traits

The Saint personality is very common today, especially among spiritually motivated people. They are trying to work their way into heaven by stretching themselves in all directions. They want to please everyone. They're the volunteers in a charity and a business. They want to be perfect in everybody's eyes, and they want to be appreciated for their tireless work. Unfortunately, all too often they are taken advantage of and thoroughly underappreciated—in many cases, even abused.

What they lack is self-love and a strong sense of self. They feel that the only way to bring safety to their environments is to make everyone around them happy, so they struggle with all their might to please. Ultimately, they assume far too much responsibility for others. Unknowingly, they violate their own boundaries and their neighbors' boundaries. Nor do they realize that they are motivated not just by the goodness of their hearts—which is considerable—but by the fear that exists inside them. Essentially, they fear that they will be blamed if people are not happy. Deep down, they believe that they are, in fact, responsible for everyone's happiness. And since this is an impossible task, they are continually failing in their own eyes and the eyes of others. In the end, Saints are continually stressed, overworked, and underappreciated. Meanwhile, all this activity is driving up dopamine, which makes them feel terrible because they do not like anxiety and would rather be comfortable at home with their families.

This brain chemistry profile is very common among adult children of alcoholics. These people were raised in families in which abuse was common and came at them at unexpected times. Alcoholic parents frequently blame their children for the parents' own faults and problems. Children, of course, are easy targets, especially for an adult's frustration and rage. Often, a child decides that the parent's unhappiness is the child's fault, and indeed the parent's blame of the child is appropriate. They think to themselves, "I'm not smart enough," or "I'm not attractive enough," or "I cannot love enough . . . Otherwise, my parents would be happy."

Meanwhile, they are often the target of unexpected abuse, which makes them fearful within their own environment. This drives up dopamine and norepinephrine, which forms the basis for a new baseline. Unfortunately, these are Satiation personalities, loving children who want very much to be close to their parents and want everyone in the family to be happy.

This very psychology, which is an adaptation to an unhealthy family environment, is brought into adulthood. As adults, Saints continue to see and react to the world as they did as children. They never developed the coping skills to deal with such stresses, and even as adults cannot effectively cope with the onslaught of so many demands. They cannot prioritize these demands, or recognize which of them should be ignored. Consequently, they are overwhelmed. Saints want satiation, but instead get continual arousal in the form of demands.

Neurochemically, the dilemma is of a Satiation personality who is extremely uncomfortable with high dopamine, but whose life is arranged to increase dopamine. This elevation of dopamine is destabilizing to the personality, throwing Saints into perpetual insecurity. That insecurity exists at the foundation of their world and causes them to constantly struggle against it.

Thus Saints are continually working hard, struggling to make the world safe for themselves and others. In the process, they can become workaholics — but not for the rewards of upward mobility, or ambition, or even money, but to create safety above all else.

Relationships

Saints desperately want close relationships and friendships, but can easily be hurt. As Satiation types, Saints want intimacy, long conversations, security, and comfort within a relationship. They are better with one on-one interactions than with a group. Their relationships are centered around emotions and the need to be close, but like all Satiation personalities, Saints can be hurt easily.

As for social situations, Saints are better with unstructured events and with those that involve less activity. The more people involved, the more activity woven into an event, and the greater the social demands, the higher the Saint's anxiety.

Saints need plenty of time for quiet self-reflection. They can easily become stressed or anxious and eventually depressed when internal stresses build up.

The opinions of others are so important that Saints can become extremely disturbed and hurt when someone does not think well of them. Trust, though very hard to establish for Saints, is a necessity for health.

Addictions and Compulsions

Saints tend to be perfectionists and to compulsively control their relationships and environment. Saints are often so overwrought that they frequently procrastinate or lose concentration. Saints often suffer from food addictions, and are particularly attracted to sweets to drive up serotonin levels. They can drink alcohol, but usually do not overindulge or drink to excess. They are rarely attracted to drugs, but if they are, the drug of choice will be marijuana or tranquilizers.

Spirituality

Saints approach spiritual life with fervor and emotion. On the other hand, they are either consciously or secretly angry at God for making life so difficult for them. They are unable to see that they themselves are causing their own problems. What they mistake for selfishness is really self-love. But since they have labeled selfishness as bad, they effectively banished it to the part of the psyche referred to as the shadow, where all that people regard as bad or evil is stored. Being selfish, taking care of oneself, knowing one's limits, recognizing one's personal responsibility for happiness—all of these are regarded by the Saint as essentially wrong, and not even to be considered. Thus Saints cut themselves off from what they need most in life: balance.

Transformation

All of this makes Saints highly vulnerable to spiritual and psychological crisis. Eventually, they either burn out or become angry and bitter. In the aftermath of this crisis, many Saints learn to integrate into their consciousness personal responsibility and the need to protect themselves. Saints finally learn boundaries, and in the process become more whole. This is the spiritual and psychological challenge facing the Saint.

The Saint's Program for Peak Performance

If you are a Saint, the bar graph below summarizes which of the techniques will work best at balancing your neurochemistry. The higher the number on the bar graph, the greater the impact that technique will have on your brain chemistry.

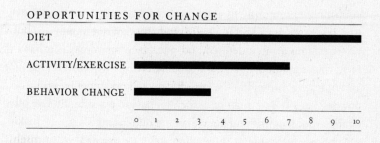

OPPORTUNITIES FOR CHANGE

DIET

ACTIVITY/EXERCISE

BEHAVIOR CHANGE

0   1   2   3   4   5   6   7   8   9   10

Behavior Change

Changing behavior will have a powerful influence on you, but it will be difficult at first because behavioral change challenges you to see life in a whole new way. The first and most difficult fact that you must incorporate into your life is that you are responsible, first and foremost, for yourself. You may also have responsibilities for your family and loved ones. The difficult truth is that there is a limit to what you can do to provide them with happiness and you must respect that limit, even honor it. You must develop a new sense of boundaries based on the real knowledge of your own limitations. Without such knowledge, you will live without borders, without balance, and without wisdom.

The establishment of boundaries based on a realistic sense of your own limits and limited responsibility for others is particularly difficult for you because you are afraid to place limits on yourself and especially on others. You must challenge that fear and explore your limits, which means you must learn to say no.

Saying no is so painful to you, yet so essential to your health, that you will be torn in two directions every time you are required to utter the word. Yet, by saying no, you will create a safer and more secure environment for yourself. At first, saying no may promote dopamine production, because it will generate some conflict within you and perhaps some anger. But as you get used to feeling your boundaries and limits, as you get used to protecting yourself, you will grow to love yourself so much more. Ultimately, defining healthy boundaries will contribute enormously to your psychological health and well-being, which is to say, it will promote the production of serotonin.

Creating a more defined and safe place for yourself in life will raise your serotonin levels. At the same time, it will lower dopamine and norepinephrine. In other words, you will no longer be sitting on a powder keg. If you maintain such behavior consistently, you will change your baseline and life will come into balance.

Meanwhile, at least three other steps are essential in your transformation. You must change your way of eating, get regular exercise, and seek spiritual counseling to establish a healthier spiritual life.

Diet

The diet for Satiation personality 1 (described in chapter 7) will do two things for you: It will increase serotonin by dramatically increasing carbohydrates in your diet. At the same time, those carbohydrates will crowd out many of the protein foods you are currently eating, which means that it will lower dopamine. Diet will have a profound effect on your neurochemistry. Meanwhile, follow these guidelines in your daily eating:

1. Make complex carbohydrates, such as whole grains, whole-grain breads, pastas, bagels, and flour products your central foods.

2. Eat lots of vegetables, especially potatoes, squash, and roots; and fruit.

3. For protein foods, eat fish, the white meat of poultry, and low-fat dairy products (if you desire them).

4. Add a complex carbohydrate snack two hours after a protein meal.

5. Avoid red meats and eggs.

6. Try to limit high-protein foods to once a day or three times a week.

7. Eat high-protein foods when you need a boost in self-confidence or personal power or when preparing for a special meeting or presentation.

8. Eat whole grains, flour products, and sweets to help you relax.

9. Avoid white sugar to prevent wide swings in blood sugar.

10. Avoid the following foods or eat them sparingly: pickled herring; pork and pork products; whole milk; most cheeses, especially cheddar, Stilton, and Camembert (high in protein and fat); ripe bananas (loaded with sugar); raisins; avocados; liver; and figs.

11. Avoid caffeine, including coffee, chocolate, and other caffeine-containing products, or use sparingly.

Activity/Exercise

Exercise is an essential part of your transformation, but it must be considered something you do for yourself that is fun. Choose the exercise program for Satiation personality 1, which is for low serotonin, high dopamine (described in chapter 8). Daily walks to work off stress and restore your sense of connectedness with your inner self are especially helpful. In addition, competitive games will give you a sense of strength and help you establish clearer boundaries between you and other people. Couple competitive games with satiation activities to achieve a balanced neurochemistry. Play tennis, basketball, or some other sport, and couple that with walking, stretching, or low-impact aerobics.

When you learn your limits, when you respect balance and boundaries, your life will open up and become truly enjoyable. What's more, the good works that you do will be more appreciated by others, in part because other people realize that you now have the capacity to say no, which makes the act of saying yes so much more valuable.

17

Type Eight

The Fire Starter

The Fire Starter is an Arousal personality with low to normal serotonin and high dopamine—which suits this type just fine. If ever there was a burning bush of a personality, it is the Fire Starter.

Personality Traits

A great many Fire Starters are blessed with some type of overwhelming talent that thoroughly shapes their lives. Often that talent is in athletics. In any case, Fire Starters are often spoiled by their magical abilities to perform heroically in whatever field they shine.

People do not necessarily have to have their talent acknowledged to be Fire Starters. Many people believe themselves to be extremely talented and carry on as if everyone recognized some special ability implicit in them. This belief may also shape the person's life as thoroughly as it might if the person were hearing cheers from audiences everywhere.

Nevertheless, most Fire Starters are acknowledged talents, and with good reason: They shine both because of their talent and their love of danger and challenge. Their arousal natures, coupled with their love of dopamine, make them take enormous risks. They place themselves in situations that others regard as too threatening or dangerous, yet these situations are exactly what draws out their talent. Somehow, they manage to perform brilliantly under the most intense of pressures, which they themselves often create. These are Arousal personalities with a love for high dopamine. They are continually looking for intense situations that raise the stakes a little higher in order to create a bigger rush, a greater risk, and thus help them shine just a little brighter. As one might expect, many actors, athletes, musicians, singers, writers, and artists are Fire Starters.

Nevertheless, what Socrates once said of the poet is also true of Fire Starters: They are controlled by the muse. Fire Starters are often thoroughly dominated by their special talent, and are only interested in the arenas in which that talent can shine. Everything outside the stage—whether it is the baseball diamond or the football field or the footlights of Broadway—is something of a letdown. The centerpiece of their lives is performing or preparing to perform. They need the intensity (read elevated dopamine) to feel alive.

Relationships

Fire Starters have relatively little interest in intimacy and close relationships, unless their mates or friends are there to cheer them on or celebrate their abilities. As members of an audience—even an audience at home—lovers, spouses, and friends are essential. Fire Starters need an audience nearly as much as they need food. On the other hand, satiation activities hold no interest for Fire Starters at all. They generally do not understand other people, nor are they particularly interested in them. Relationships must have some type of goal, usually one that leads them a little closer to the realization of their ambition. In order for social situations to work, they must be structured and grounded in some form of activity.

At the bottom of nearly all Fire Starters' problems with relationships is their inability to establish a relationship with their deeper selves. Because they do not know themselves outside their special abilities, they are unable to express their deeper desires, their wounds, and their more intimate selves. Just as they are unable to gain access to themselves, they are also unable to become intimate with others.

Instead, they want praise and adulation, never fully accepting that such love will fade the minute they stop performing at their current levels. In other words, they receive the most conditional of all love, which will eventually be pulled out from under them and cause tremendous pain. Nevertheless, while their talents are shining, they evaluate people in the most simplistic of terms: "What have you done for me lately?"

Because of their high dopamine and their need for dedication, Fire Starters are often very demanding sexually. Sex plays a central part in their relationships and they often evaluate a relationship on how good the sex is. High dopamine and norepinephrine make the Fire Starter hungry for arousal and experience.

Fire Starters are frequently immature in many areas of their lives. They often have little interest in academics, unless that is where their talents lie. Many Fire Starters were singled out as having learning disabilities as children—not so much because they were unintelligent, but because they had little or no interest in school. Their dopamine was too high to allow them to sit still or pay attention to a teacher for very long. Many have trouble focusing on details. They see things in the broadest terms, in part because they are people of action. They are doers, not thinkers. Give them a general idea of what you want accomplished and let them loose. But don't be surprised if what you end up with looks nothing like what you originally had in mind. Fire Starters are controlled by the muse, not by mere mortals.

Fire Starters are great beginners but lousy finishers. They get bored quickly and move on to more exciting situations or relationships. If you tell a Fire Starter that he should ride his bicycle two miles a day for the entire summer, he'll get really excited and ride his bike twenty miles the first day—and never get back on the bike again. He's bored. The bike no longer interests him. He runs intensely hot at first and then turns cold, disinterested, bored. Whatever excited him initially about a plan or relationship may not hold the least bit of interest a day later.

On an unconscious but very visceral level, Fire Starters have decided that it is essential to be a slave to their talents in order to bring them to their full flowering. It's as if they are dominated by one dimension of their being, a dimension they must serve in order to fully realize its potential. When the light of that talent begins to dim or goes out, however, they are often thrown into crisis. This is the point at which Fire Starters are most capable of change. It is also the moment of greatest danger.

Addictions and Compulsions

Fire Starters are highly vulnerable to addictions and compulsions— anything that dramatically raises dopamine and provides a rush of arousal. Sexual conquest and addiction is very common. So is cocaine addiction.

Cocaine can satisfy any one of several needs. First, it increases dopamine dramatically, which enhances performance and makes Fire Starters even better at what they normally excel at. Second, it gives them the kind of rush that they love and otherwise can get only from intense situations. However, cocaine is used by many Fire Starters after they have begun to doubt their abilities, or when their abilities have started to wane. Cocaine then becomes a way to restore performance to its former heights. It is a way to reexperience the lofty excitation that their sheer ability gave them in their youth. As so many Fire Starters have learned, however, cocaine first ruins your life and then it kills you.

Once Fire Starters are addicted, it is very difficult for them to change. They fear that without the drug or compulsion, they will not be able to perform at the level once reached without external support. Anyone who seeks to change a Fire Starter will have quite a job. They are unreflective about their behavior and expect others to praise them relentlessly, even after a single day of improved behavior. "I didn't do any cocaine today," a Fire Starter will say with a look of expectation, as if she had just saved the President of the United States from certain death. "Isn't that great!"

Spirituality

Fire Starters do not indulge much in self-reflection, nor are they overly given to contemplating their relationship to the universe. Yet spirituality holds a secret interest for them when they can slow down long enough to look up into the night's sky with wonder. Fire Starters become more self-reflective with age. Mellowing helps them to see life in a broader perspective. At that point, they are far more open to spiritual counsel and literature. The key for Fire Starters to open up spiritually is to slow down and learn to enjoy more satiation activities and a satiation approach to life. Ironically, there are Fire Starter ministers. These people tend to be so charismatic that people flock to them as if they were movie stars. Fire Starter ministers often become gurus to their followers. Unfortunately, those types of relationships often end after severe conflict of one type or another.

The Fire Starter's Program for Peak Performance

If you are a Fire Starter, the bar graph below summarizes the kinds of techniques that will be most effective in changing your brain chemistry. The higher the number on the bar graph, the greater the impact that technique will have on your neurochemistry.

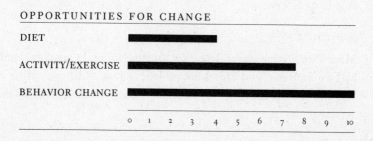

OPPORTUNITIES FOR CHANGE

Behavior Change

You are an extreme personality; one side of your being is well developed and the other side is somewhat neglected. In order to optimize your brain chemistry and make it possible for you to function at far higher levels and within a much wider context, you must create balance in your life. This means developing the more receptive, open, loving, and intimate side of your being.

The best way to do this is by opening up to the needs and sensitivities of another human being. As with all people, love changes the Fire Starter. However, you need a particularly strong person to direct you away from your preoccupation with yourself. You must awaken to the consequences of your behavior on the person you truly care about. This simple awareness can be the basis for a remarkable transformation. It is based on the recognition that you are part of an interdependent world in which all members count on each other for support and nourishment.

In terms of brain chemistry, this awareness and the actions that support it raise serotonin and lower dopamine. Such behaviors require that you get to know another person and, indeed, yourself. Intimacy, the thing you may be most afraid of, becomes the basis for restoring balance and broadening your view of life. The effects of such behavior will be to slow you down, balance your otherwise high-tension lifestyle, and allow you to enjoy your relationships in a new and fulfilling way. You will be amazed at the joys and rewards and growth that emerge from intimacy with those you love.

For all these reasons, behavioral change can have the most powerful influence on your brain chemistry, and holds the key to your long-term happiness.

Activity/Exercise

Many Fire Starters are athletes (the professional ranks are dominated by Fire Starters), and others are athletic actors. Still, you can find Fire Starters in virtually all professions—they are usually the stars.

Whether you are an athletic or nonathletic Fire Starter, you will be able to balance your neurochemistry most effectively by engaging in satiation exercises. Unfortunately, these tend to be your least favorite exercises.

Fire Starters love competition and high-intensity athletics, but you are able to balance your neurochemistry best by walking, gentle bicycling, stretching, and low-impact aerobics (see the list of exercises for satiation in chapter 8). These exercises raise serotonin and lower dopamine, causing you to feel more relaxed, more focused, and better able to slow your life down. By doing these exercises, you will be able to open up to the other side of your being, the more receptive, gentle, and loving side. (See the list of satiation exercises in chapter 8.)

Diet

Optimizing your brain chemistry means restoring balance to your life. The best way to do that with diet is to include more satiation foods, such as complex carbohydrates from whole grains and flour products. You should adopt the diet for Arousal personality 2 (described in chapter 7), and follow these guidelines:

1. Reduce or eliminate all forms of red meat and eggs from your diet.
2. Rely on fish, chicken, beans, and tofu for your protein needs.
3. Eat these high-protein foods whenever you need to perform or feel you need to be stronger or more aggressive.
4. Reduce your intake of Healthy Zone and Occasional Zone animal foods to four times per week. After two to three weeks, reduce animal foods again to three times per week.
5. Include a whole-grain food or dish at every meal. This will boost your serotonin levels significantly and reduce dopamine-boosting protein foods.
6. Snack on whole grains and foods made of whole-grain flour (rice cakes, cookies, popcorn, pastries, raisin bread, others).

7. Eliminate or significantly reduce all caffeinated beverages and foods, such as coffee and chocolate.

8. Significantly reduce or eliminate all whole-milk products and hard cheeses, such as cheddar, Swiss, and others.

Fire Starters often gain the kind of balance that makes healthy relationships possible when they awaken to the love of another human being, or when their careers as athletes or stars have peaked or passed. Such events—either great love or the passing of your career—can be very difficult for you, in part because you only recognize yourself as a star and not as an equal or a partner in a mutually satisfying relationship. Eventually, life forces all Fire Starters—even you!—to come down from Olympus and walk among the mortals. Ironically, such humbling can restore balance and equilibrium to your life and opens you up to truly lasting rewards. Careers pass, great moments fade, but, as the poet has said, love abides forever.

18

Type Nine

The Mediator

Most Mediators are Satiation personalities with balanced brain chemistry—normal serotonin and relatively stable dopamine. Because of their stable dopamine, Mediators do not struggle to stand out or get attention. They do not cause a lot of conflict and they are not overly aggressive.

Personality Traits

Mediators are highly flexible, capable of understanding, appreciating, and working with a wide variety of people and viewpoints. For this reason, I call them Mediators, because that is the role they so often play in social and professional situations and group dynamics.

Remarkably, Mediators tend to have an intuitive gift for balancing their neurochemistry. They self-medicate well. When they are feeling depressed, they somehow know the kinds of foods to eat and the exercises to perform. They also avoid the kinds of foods that will lower serotonin or raise dopamine (namely high protein). Like everyone, Mediators need to elevate serotonin when they get depressed, but they are fairly balanced in both serotonin and dopamine, so that extremes of depression and anxiety are not particularly common.

Mediators have a kind of quiet intelligence. They focus on issues, concentrate on the details, and come up with solutions without raising the flag and wanting horns to blare (all high-serotonin characteristics). They are excellent problem solvers, highly creative in an understated way. They also are good with follow-through. Mediators are plodders (another high-serotonin quality). They don't get pushed around by a lot of internal stresses and anxiety (a characteristic of balanced dopamine). Hence they are able to concentrate on issues over long periods of time and see them through to resolution. They are good team players; they take a practical approach to problem-solving; and they synthesize many different points of view into the group's solution. They respond best to short-term goals, to which they will dedicate themselves thoroughly.

Because of their intelligence and flexibility, Mediators often find themselves as executives and leaders within groups or corporations, or as members of the legal profession. Whatever their profession, they are rarely the stars. Rather, they are the people the stars count on to help them find solutions.

Some of this may suggest that Mediators are repressed. One might speculate that they may be trying to fit into some perfect image of the background figure with all the answers. Frankly, there are many repressed people trying to be Mediator types, but true Mediators love life, are full of humor, and don't hide their problems or suffering. True Mediators are real people, with real problems, but blessed with a balanced approach to life. They are not overly ambitious; they are practical people, with practical goals that are well within reach. Because of their balanced view of people and situations, they tend to be promoted within a group or company and naturally find themselves in positions of authority. People naturally trust them, because they seem to judge fairly.

Relationships

As Satiation personalities, Mediators love intimacy, family, and long-term relationships. They prefer calm settings so that interaction is enhanced. Being respected is very important to Mediators, though they don't pursue it openly. Mediators want to be helpful to others; but unlike the Saints, Mediators know their limits and respect the fact that they cannot be all things to all people.

Mediators also need quiet times to be by themselves to self-reflect. As with other Satiation types, a great deal of excitement can quickly cause anxiety for the Mediator.

Spirituality

Mediators take a quiet, internal approach to spirituality. They approach spiritual matters from both emotional and intellectual perspectives. They tend to be good listeners, they support others, and they are not particularly critical of other people. They tend to shy away from big displays of emotion, however.

The Mediator's Program for Peak Performance

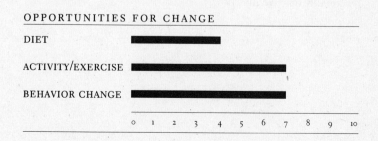

OPPORTUNITIES FOR CHANGE

DIET	
ACTIVITY/EXERCISE	
BEHAVIOR CHANGE	

0 1 2 3 4 5 6 7 8 9 10

As a Mediator, you have an intuitive sense of balance and know how to adjust your neurochemistry to maintain that balance. Therefore no one technique will have a more significant impact on health than any other.

Diet

The diet for Satiation personality 1, which boosts serotonin, will work fine for you.

Activity/Exercise

The exercise program for Satiation personality 2, for low serotonin and normal dopamine, comes the closest to being helpful to the Mediator, but you should do whatever exercises you are currently enjoying.

The Mediator is not the perfect personality type. In comparison with some of the other types—especially the more dynamic personalities, such as the Awakening Warrior, Boatman, or Armored Knight—the Mediator appears staid, and not a little understated. Indeed, without every personality type our world would be very dull. The unique characteristic of Mediators is that they have an innate ability to balance their brain chemistry, at least within certain limits. When under routine or higher levels of stress, Mediators have an intuitive understanding of which foods and behavioral traits will restore their sense of equilibrium.

That ability is something most of us can develop, no matter what personality type we may be.

Epilogue: Your Inner State and the Outer World

Serotonin, Dopamine, and the Spiritual Crisis

Many people today express concern about the powerful media images of violence, horror, and sex that all of us—especially our children—are exposed to each day. Few, however, can articulate these concerns clearly, because no one has found a way to objectively show the effects these images are having on our collective and individual psyches.

Hence we find ourselves talking in vague generalities about the "absence of values," or the need to establish "family values." We use broad terms like the "spiritual crisis" in America and the world today. Unfortunately, such terms—however well intended—are far too amorphous to create consensus or galvanize rational actions, and many people experience the emotion-filled rhetoric as personally threatening.

I believe that we can find the functional vocabulary we are looking for in the neurochemistry model, which provides a clear and objective way of describing the effects such images are having on brain chemistry and psychology. I call these effects the "acceleration syndrome": the continual need to boost dopamine in order to give us a sense of being alive.

The world we live in is becoming increasingly addicted to the gas-pedal neurotransmitters. We need more and more stimulation in order to maintain the sense of excitement and arousal that they provide.

At bottom, our problems stem from a neurochemical imbalance: Most people today are deficient in serotonin and excessive in dopamine and norepinephrine—low on satiation and high on arousal—and this imbalance appears to be growing. We are less and less calm; we have a growing inability to concentrate and focus on the deeper aspects of problems. As a society, we sleep less than we used to, and for many the hours we do sleep are restless and shallow. It is harder and harder to achieve a sense of well-being. Many millions of us are depressed. We have lost a sense of direction and faith in the future. All of these feelings are symptomatic of low serotonin.

At the same time, our society is increasingly restless, afraid, and violent. Violence occurs at younger ages and it permeates every aspect of our society. There are very few safe places in America any more. These developments are all symptoms of excess dopamine and norepinephrine.

This underlying neurochemical imbalance is reshaping our world. It informs our beliefs about the state of our world and changes our expectations about the future. Since we act on our beliefs and expectations, our actions are the fruit of the serotonin-dopamine imbalance. In short, we are motivated increasingly by fear.

Previous generations, more richly endowed with serotonin, were able to express a greater patience with each other's foibles and mistakes. Today people are shooting at each other on the freeway because one driver offended another. I do not have to list all the crimes and craziness in our world to make my point.

In general, we can say that arousal is up. Violent and arousing images are pervasive in our society, and far more than ever before. Local television news depends on vivid images of violence to maintain their ratings. Video games present increasingly violent images in order to sustain sales. Sex is used ever more graphically as a sales tool. All of this takes place against the age-old tapestry of war, famine, floods, earthquakes, and assorted other tragedies that, thanks to television news, seem to be taking place in our own homes. Much is made today of the "global village," the shrinking of our world, thanks to the "revolution" (a dopamine-boosting word) in communications technology. And indeed, many wonderful things are happening by virtue of this global communications network. Yet somehow we are left with the impression that most of the news is bad.

The use of violence, sex, and horror as sales tools is predicated on consumer demand. The media would be out of business in no time were it not for the fact that sex and violence sell. The public wants these images. Otherwise, we would turn off the television set; we would not patronize films; we would demand that certain types of advertising not grace our magazines or billboards. The public is as much to blame as anyone, we are told.

Presentations such as the one I am offering always come down to this point, and very often end here as well. How else are we to feel but that we are "bad" people or "sick" people to want such things? Such labels prevent us from examining ourselves and the problems we face. They force us to rationalize away our guilt by saying that it isn't me who looks at or attends such films, and so on. Rationalizing merely keeps us from addressing the problem head-on.

What is that problem? In a nutshell, we are increasingly addicted to experiences that arouse, which means we are addicted to thoughts, images, foods, and behaviors that boost dopamine and norepinephrine. Protein-rich foods, such as meat, eggs, and some dairy products; caffeine; violent and sexual media images; various pharmaceutical and recreational drugs, such as cocaine—these are just a handful of the ways we get our dopamine rush each day. Drug addiction, so widespread today, is actually a metaphor for our society's current condition. The baseline neurochemistry is changing so that serotonin is lower and dopamine is higher. Unfortunately, the impact of this imbalance in favor of dopamine has its most profound effect on the young.

Several years ago, I began to advise a high school student named Jessie. Jessie came from a family of highly active people who moved from one home to another several times when Jessie was young. As Jessie grew up, he became chronically anxious and tense. He dealt with his tension by overeating and watching a lot of television. He also went to the movies quite often and became enamored with action-packed, violent films and horror movies. In addition to anxiety, Jessie had low self-esteem. Deep inside himself, he didn't believe he was much good at anything. People urged Jessie to get out and exercise. Become more active like your parents, people told him. In fact, Jessie tried to get involved in sports and attempted several exercise programs, but he couldn't stick to any of them. Eventually, he just gave up and kept eating and watching TV and going to the movies.

Finally, his father brought him to me for a neurochemical evaluation. I found that he was a Satiation personality with low serotonin and excessively high levels of dopamine and norepinephrine, which caused his anxiety and tension. Television helped him relax part of the time (generally a satiation activity), but many of the shows he watched—and especially the movies he attended—were highly arousing (dopamine and norepinephrine boosters). He was constantly being aroused beyond his tolerance for dopamine and norepinephrine by images on television and in films. This made him anxious, tense, and afraid. It also kept him returning to satiation activities—sitting on the couch watching television with a bowl of food in front of him.

The first thing I did was have Jessie eat foods that raised his serotonin levels—namely complex carbohydrates—and lowered his dopamine-norepinephrine levels. This meant that he had to restrict his protein intake. Jessie ate lots of brown rice, noodles and bread and some sweets; he also ate low-fat sources of protein daily, but he couldn't snack on pizza and other high-fat, high-protein foods. I also encouraged his family to restrict his television watching and movie going. He had to limit the television shows and films, and he had to avoid horror movies or excessively violent films. All of these changes raised his serotonin levels, which boosted his confidence and self-esteem and lowered his dopamine and norepinephrine, which reduced his anxiety.

The reduction in television watching had a remarkable impact on Jessie. He was now in a situation in which he couldn't just turn on the TV and get his usual dopamine and norepinephrine rush. He had to find something else to drive up his dopamine and norepinephrine levels, so he started playing sports and became more active.

Over a two-year period, Jessie made a remarkable transformation. He lowered his weight and became a more focused and determined young man. He doesn't have the same low self-esteem as he had, nor does he have the anxiety.

Jessie was addicted to extremes of arousal, which he dealt with by high doses of satiation. His dopamine-serotonin imbalance combined to create a high-fat, low-exercise lifestyle that would eventually have killed him. Unfortunately, there are millions of Jessies out there today, and consequently the individual Jessies do not stand out.

Obesity is increasing in America, especially among the young. Parents lament the fact that their kids aren't active, but they're like all the other kids. Children are dealing with arousal and its accompanying nervous and muscular tension by indulging in satiation, which usually means sweet and high-fat foods. This is only natural. Our society is driving many children inward because of the intense arousal they must endure. Other children respond by acting out those aroused states. Meanwhile, we feed these children enormous amounts of high-protein, high-fat foods, which arouses them further. Their next blast of protein—in the form of a "happy meal"—is as close as the nearest Mac-Donald's. Increasingly, the American family thinks of Wendy's, Burger

King, and MacDonald's as a standard source of food each week. Many Americans, especially the young, eat at such places every day.

Very often, arousal is taking place while people are sitting. They are witnessing images or eating foods that send dopamine levels soaring. Yet they are passive witnesses of these images, they are resting consumers. The result is that energy, muscles, and respiration are not being utilized. Dopamine is not being burned up. It is increased and stored, waiting for its moment to trigger some type of behavior. Meanwhile, serotonin falls. The combination causes anxiety and depression, which is a volatile mix that very often leads to violence.

Our children are proving the brain chemistry model, but in reverse. Rather than biochemistry determining thoughts and behaviors, images and thoughts are changing their biochemistry. Many people think when they hear those words that I am talking about something good, about a way to escape depression or anxiety. But the mechanisms work in both directions. We can fill our lives with negative images and thoughts and thereby change our biochemistry for the worse. By pumping up dopamine and norepinephrine levels, we are turning our children into arousal junkies.

When scientists examine the effects of this imbalance on animals, they see very graphically the kinds of behaviors we are witnessing in our society today. At the University of California at Los Angeles (UCLA), scientists have found that monkeys have a distinct social hierarchy, in which the highest-ranking males have the highest levels of serotonin, while the lowest-ranking have the lowest serotonin levels. The lower-ranking monkeys with low serotonin (and thus relatively higher dopamine and norepinephrine) are the most prone to violence. Indeed, as I pointed out earlier, human studies have confirmed that people with low serotonin and high dopamine react in much the same way: With higher than average hostility and violence.

Ironically, animal studies and human experience suggest that these neurochemical conditions and behaviors can be changed. At UCLA, scientists have discovered that when one of the lower-ranking monkeys begins to move up the social hierarchy, his serotonin levels increase, as well. Apparently, the rise in status *causes* the monkey's serotonin to increase, which makes him more relaxed, focused, and calm. The opposite also takes place: When a dominant monkey falls from his lofty position, his serotonin levels fall.

Research on humans has shown that the officers of college fraternities have higher serotonin levels than the average fraternity student. The experience of people who take serotonin-boosting drugs, such as Prozac, has shown that with higher serotonin comes greater self-esteem and less likelihood of violence.

Do love and status trigger increases in serotonin? Surely they do. But we must consider the importance of the baseline and its resistance to change. The love must be consistent, and the elevation in status must remain in place long enough to alter the baseline. Then the change is made.

None of these transformations would be possible if we were irrevocably caught in a biological cycle in which habits gave rise to neurochemical events that reinforced habits. We would be caught in our own sameness, until whatever harmful side effects accompanied such behavior ended up killing us. Yet we know that many people make radical changes in beliefs, outlook, and behavior. People overcome this imbalance and are restored to health. Alcoholics, compulsive gamblers, and drug addicts overcome addictions. People experience true spiritual and religious conversions. Many stop behaviors that are hurting themselves and others; some of these same people start whole new ways of living that are enriching and life-supportive. They contribute to the common good. Our world is kept sane by those who make such conversions, and by those whose behavior flows from life-supporting values each day. It isn't just from our literature that we draw hope. There have been millions of real-life Ebenezer Scrooges, just as there have been millions of real-life Macbeths. People make dramatic changes. Many of these transformations are for the individual and collective good; others are not.

The brain chemistry model instructs us objectively on how to make positive change, using food, behavior, images, and thoughts.

When insightful people talk about the spiritual crisis we face, they often say that Americans are searching for meaning. The old belief systems required an almost unquestioned faith and acceptance of certain precepts. Today, many people need to understand those precepts at a deeper level. Deeper meanings exist and certainly will be found by seekers. One way to find such meaning in the religious and spiritual traditions of the past is to apply the brain chemistry model. When we do that, we see an underlying wisdom that did indeed support and nurture human growth and happiness.

If we examine the spiritual traditions of virtually every people, we find that many basic tenets are the same. The common values among all religions are love of God, love of self, and love of others; compassion for one's fellow humans; adherence to truth; and avoidance of certain behaviors, such as killing and stealing. When we look at the basic tools that are meant to encourage growth and happiness, we find great similarities: meditation and prayer, deep self-reflection, remorse for wrongdoing, speaking the truth from one's heart. An examination of the spiritual life of traditional people in the East and West reveals a common approach to daily life, including faith in the Creator, daily prayer, simple living and eating.

When looked at from a brain chemistry model, we recognize that spiritual life promotes high serotonin and low dopamine. Biochemically, spiritual life promotes greater peace, greater concentration, more receptivity, slower neurotransmission, less violence, and less arousal. It does precisely the opposite of what our society is doing today.

We can draw many conclusions from such information, but one thing is radiantly clear: We suffer from a spiritual crisis in part because our lifestyles have created a neurochemistry and behaviors that are essentially self-destructive.

We possess the power to change our lives for the better. All we need is to learn how to use that power. The tools for transformation that many of us are looking for—perhaps all of us are looking for—lie in a spiritual life. They reside in the serotonin-boosting practices, such as prayer, meditation, faith, simple living, and simple eating.

Many people argue that we should all have greater reverence for life and respect for our fellow humans, and that this would take care of our social ills. But these values cannot be experienced as long as so many of us are neurochemically imbalanced. Reverence for life and respect for others are the fruits of a balanced brain chemistry. They exist because healthy lifestyles and healthy thoughts exist first.

The brain chemistry model takes us above the discussion of "good" people and "bad" people. It helps us to see that at bottom we are all the same, though each of us is struggling with different degrees of imbalance. Our society cannot be transformed until we have established a greater sense of balance, especially neurochemical balance. And that balance can only be achieved by using the tools offered to us by our spiritual and religious traditions.

This is part of the wisdom that lies below the surface of these teachings: Among other things, they are inherently health producing for individuals and society.

The secret to making them work for us lies in consistency. It takes consistent behavior to change your baseline neurochemistry, which in turn will change your inner state and your outer world. People do it every day.

Thus we begin each day with the power to alter our brain chemistries for a day and for a lifetime. To a great extent, we can choose the kinds of activities we engage in, the foods we eat, and the images and environments that we are exposed to. In this way, we can significantly raise the level of serotonin in the brain, control our soaring dopamine, and in the process, create a better world.

Robertson Institute Performance Enhancement Program

If you are interested in receiving a more detailed neurochemical evaluation and performance plan, we offer you the Robertson Performance Enhancement Program.

Robertson Institute developed this program over the years to help tailor an enhancement program for you. This program will help you to:

think more clearly

react more quickly

overcome stress and anxiety

recover quickly from a negative situation

function more effectively and efficiently

become more consistent and effective

Additionally, this results in:

enhanced interpersonal skills

improved problem-solving ability

increased self-esteem

a fuller, more productive, and happier life

You will receive a report that will tailor a diet, exercise and activity, behavioral, and spiritual program for you. You will also receive an audiotape describing the concepts that you will need to know to enhance your performance. This program requires you to complete the following Performance Enhancement Survey.

Turn to page 241 for payment instructions and coupon.

Instructions for Completing the Survey

1. Please complete all information on the top of the answer sheet, including your name, address, and phone number.
2. Take your time and read all the questions thoroughly.
3. Your answers should reflect your feelings over the past year rather than over the last few days or weeks, unless otherwise stated.
4. Please answer every question.
5. If you are not sure of an answer, choose the closest "true" or "false" answer.
6. If a question doesn't pertain to you or you can't determine if it is true or false, answer it "false."
7. There are no wrong answers, good answers, or bad answers, just honest answers. Please be honest
8. After completing the survey, please send your completed answer sheet along with payment to:

> Robertson Institute, Ltd.
> Testing Division
> 3555 Pierce St.
> Saginaw, MI 48604

Robertson Institute Performance Enhancement Survey

1. I prefer being alone.
2. I am a "down" person, or somewhat depressed.
3. One or more of my brothers, sisters, parents, or grandparents now have or have had arthritis or stiffness in their joints. (If you are adopted, answer this question "false.")
4. I often feel angry.
5. I spend money or buy things when I am "down," angry, or nervous.
6. I participate in group activities that have consistent guidelines and provide emotional fulfillment.
7. I watch television or read more than fifteen hours a week.
8. I find it hard to have a comfortable relationship with other people.
9. My friends or family have confronted me about spending too much time working at my job.
10. I now have difficulty remembering things I used to be able to remember easily.
11. I have become violent in situations where I was not threatened with violence.
12. It bothers me when someone does something better than I do.
13. I watch television, movies, or videos more than four hours daily, at least four days a week.
14. I feel that many people dislike me.
15. One or more of my brothers, sisters, parents, or grandparents now have or have had high blood pressure. (If you are adopted, answer this question "false.")
16. One or more of my brothers, sisters, parents, or grandparents now have or have had Alzheimer's disease or early senility. (If you are adopted, answer this question "false.")
17. I have recently experienced at least one of the four following conditions: chest pains, shortness of breath, blue fingernails, or dizziness when I stand up.
18. I have trouble being with people because I feel insecure.
19. I enjoy gambling.
20. One or more of my children may have a problem with alcoholism, gambling, drug addiction, or overeating. (If you have no children, answer this question "false.")
21. I continue to eat even after I am full.
22. I have lost more than ten pounds in thirty days without dieting.
23. People have told me that I work too much.

24. I prefer to spend time with a small group of people rather than a large group of people.

25. I am more comfortable knowing lots of people than having a few close friends.

26. I should "slow down" because I feel there is no need to push myself so fast or to do the exciting things I do.

27. During this past year, I have felt more muscle weakness.

28. During this past year, I have experienced changes in my desire or need for sex.

29. I watch exciting movies or videos or play computer games more than fifteen hours a week.

30. I experience ringing in my ears.

31. To help me relax, I have used medication, alcohol, or some other substance.

32. I experience a significant change in my mood at least three times a week.

33. When I am frustrated, angry, or stressed, I eat, even though I am not hungry.

34. When I am with people in a social setting, I am usually one of the last to leave.

35. I enjoy strenuous exercise about two times a week.

36. I dislike exercise.

37. When I am stressed or anxious, I like sexual activities to help me calm down.

38. One to three of my brothers, sisters, parents, or grandparents has a problem with alcoholism, gambling, drug addiction, or overeating. (If you are adopted, answer this question "false.")

39. I am fearful or insecure.

40. Even a small amount of anxiety makes me feel uncomfortable.

41. I have trouble getting started on projects that need to be completed.

42. Four or more of my biological aunts, uncles, or cousins have a problem with alcoholism, gambling, drug addiction, or overeating. (If you are adopted, answer this question "false.")

43. I like substances, behaviors, or activities that give me a "lift" or make me feel better.

44. I prefer highly competitive, goal-oriented activities over those that involve quiet self-reflection.

45. I become defensive when people question my judgment.

46. I like exercise that tones my muscles more than exercise that makes me perspire.

47. I watch television or videos, go to the movies, or listen to music or tapes more than fifteen hours per week.

48. People have told me that I clean or organize my home, office, or possessions too much.
49. I struggle with procrastination.
50. I have been hospitalized or have had medication prescribed for depression or "feeling down."
51. I often spend more than I earn in a month.
52. I often take part in activities that involve high risk, such as white-water rafting, mountain climbing, or driving fast cars.
53. I like to socialize with large groups of people.
54. I find myself trying to control people and situations when I get nervous or stressed.
55. I usually don't get anxious or nervous in social settings.
56. I am a loner.
57. I have gambled (including making risky financial investments) despite financial difficulties.
58. I have trouble sleeping through the night, even if not interrupted, at least four times a week.
59. I can confront people easily when I feel they have done me wrong.
60. I watch television, read, or meditate less than five hours a week.
61. I accept criticism well.
62. I watch action-oriented or competitive sports programs at least fifteen hours a week.
63. I have been more than thirty pounds overweight.
64. I get depressed or feel down if I don't do my best.
65. I have seen things that were not real when I was not drinking alcohol or taking drugs.
66. I am more than fifty pounds overweight.
67. I like being with others more than being alone.
68. I like groups, including religious groups, that have standards, rules, or codes of behavior.
69. I experience pounding in my head, headaches, or sinus pain at least twice a week.
70. When I am depressed or feel down, I feel like I have to accomplish something to make me feel better.
71. When I feel down, I may use drugs, medications, or alcohol to help me feel better.
72. When I am with a group of people, I lose energy the longer I am with them.
73. I feel depressed or down when I am not accomplishing something.
74. I have recently begun to forget people, places, and things.

75. I buy things that I don't need, even when I feel I can't afford them.
76. I have difficulty in focusing my eyes or I often see double.
77. I have a problem with controlling people or situations.
78. I like risky activities such as speeding, mountain climbing, hang gliding, or racing.
79. I use sexual activities to make me feel better when I am down.
80. I participate in risky activities, in spite of having been injured while doing them in the past.
81. I fear people, places, or things.
82. I am more than thirty pounds but less than fifty pounds overweight.
83. When I disagree with someone, I usually remain silent.
84. I have a difficult time remaining friends with people who disagree with me.
85. I have trouble getting to sleep, even when I feel tired, at least four times weekly.
86. I am stressed or nervous.
87. I am a very calm person.
88. When I feel stressed or nervous, I drink alcohol to make me feel better.
89. I experience diarrhea or nausea frequently.
90. I drink alcoholic beverages to give me energy when I feel down.
91. I have an irregular or rapid heart rate, or perspire, without exercising.
92. I prefer to watch movies, videos, or television programs that relax me over action, horror, or violent movies, videos, or television programs.
93. I usually spend my free time alone.
94. I now have or have had seizures or convulsions.
95. I have recently felt a general tiredness.
96. I would like several sexual partners.
97. I crave sweets, carbohydrates, or other sugar-based products when I am nervous, stressed, depressed, or angry.
98. I have trouble expressing my true feelings to those I care about.
99. I drink alcoholic beverages when I become depressed.
100. I usually will drink alcoholic beverages when I am with people in a social setting, if it is available.
101. I have been hospitalized or have had medication prescribed for anxiety or nervousness.
102. One of my brothers, sisters, parents, or grandparents now has or has had cancer. (If you are adopted, answer this question "false.")
103. I prefer to do relaxing activities alone rather than be with a large group of people.
104. I prefer mild exercise to strenuous exercise.

105. I feel the need to clean my room, apartment, or home when I am depressed, angry, or nervous.
106. I am unable to relax when my room, apartment, or home needs simple cleaning.
107. One or more of my brothers, sisters, parents, or grandparents now have or have had epilepsy or convulsions. (If you are adopted, answer this question "false.")
108. I usually don't do things as well as I want to.
109. When I make a small mistake, I experience mood swings.
110. I have gained more than ten pounds in thirty days.
111. I prefer exercise that makes my heart beat faster over mild exercise.
112. I find myself feeling uncomfortable when things don't go the way I want them to.
113. I am angry.
114. When I make a small mistake, it takes me a while to forget about it.
115. I work more than sixty hours a week on a consistent basis.
116. My violent behavior or temper has caused my relationships to suffer.
117. I crave sweets, carbohydrates, or sugar-based products when I am nervous or stressed.
118. I participate in quieting activities to relax myself.
119. When I am asked to participate in activities where there is a winner, I feel nervous.
120. I need the approval of others or I get depressed.
121. It takes a great deal of frustration or conflict to make me feel nervous or stressed.
122. I purchase lottery tickets or bet on sporting events.
123. I usually watch movies, videos, or television programs or play computer games with action or excitement.
124. I experience significant mood swings on a daily basis.
125. I feel excited or good about myself when I gamble.
126. I am an angry person.
127. I now am or have been overweight.
128. I am stressed.
129. I use sex to relieve my frustrations or stress.
130. I am now or have been underweight.
131. I get bored having sex with the same person after a while.
132. I get constipated frequently.
133. I have taken prescribed medication or used alcohol or drugs to make me feel better.

134. I have trouble staying awake during the day.
135. I do not drink alcohol, use drugs, or take prescribed medication.
136. I would rather use alcohol in a quiet setting than in a social setting. (If you don't drink, answer "false.")
137. Quiet activities relax me.
138. When I drink alcohol it gives me a calming feeling.
139. I watch noncompetitive programs or events at least fifteen hours a week.
140. I have trouble urinating, have pain when I urinate, or have frequent urination.
141. I often wake up earlier than I would like.
142. I am an optimistic person.
143. I enjoy activities that require a lot of energy and excitement.
144. One or more of my brothers, sisters, parents, or grandparents are or have been more than twenty pounds but less than fifty pounds overweight. (If you are adopted, answer this question "false.")
145. I often have nasal or sinus congestion.
146. I am a positive person.
147. I enjoy spending time with a small group of people talking and sharing my feelings.
148. I worry about my health because of the amount of stress I am feeling.
149. One or more of my brothers, sisters, parents, or grandparents now have or have had heart problems. (If you are adopted, answer this question "false.")
150. I get stressed or nervous rather easily.
151. When I make a mistake and am confronted, I try to avoid the issue or make up excuses.
152. One or more of my brothers, sisters, parents, or grandparents are or have been at least fifty pounds overweight. (If you are adopted, answer this question "false.")
153. I have become violent and struck someone close to me more than one time.
154. I enjoy competitive activities.
155. I prefer a few close relationships to knowing a lot of people.
156. I have been convicted of a legal wrongdoing or put on probation at my work because of my personal actions.
157. I enjoy watching or participating in violent activities.
158. I crave sweets, carbohydrates, or sugar-based products when I am down or depressed.
159. People close to me complain about my procrastination.
160. I drink alcohol or use mood-altering substances at least four times a week.
161. I prefer activities in which I can be an active participant over activities in which I am a spectator.

162. I prefer activities in which I can be a spectator over activities in which I am an active participant.

163. I have had hallucinations, or heard voices or sounds, when I was not drinking alcohol or using drugs.

164. I watch television, movies, or videos more than fifteen hours a week.

165. Food, alcohol, or other substances, including prescription drugs, that decrease my nervousness or stress make me feel better.

166. People do not support me or believe in me.

167. I find it difficult to concentrate because of my stress levels.

168. I have recently had a loss of appetite.

169. One of my brothers, sisters, parents, or grandparents now has or has had diabetes. (If you are adopted, answer this question "false.")

170. I tend to spend less time with people who disagree with me.

171. I have tried to lose weight in the past and failed.

172. I prefer to bet on a game in order to add excitement.

173. Do you suffer from any of the following: addiction, overweight, underweight, depression, anxiety, mood swings?

174. Do you have a history of any of the following: heart disease, high blood pressure, high cholesterol, diabetes, other major medical condition?

175. According to your doctor, is your overall health excellent or above average?

176. Are you an active person under the age of forty-five years, with no family history of heart disease and no medical conditions?

177. Are you a semi-active or active person under the age of sixty-five years with no medical conditions?

178. Are you relatively inactive or do you have medical conditions that will interfere with your health?

179. Do you have restrictions in your diet?

180. Do you have restrictions on your exercise or activity?

Robertson Institute
Performance Enhancement Survey Answer Sheet

NAME _____ DATE _____

STREET ADDRESS _____

CITY _____ STATE _____ ZIP CODE _____

COUNTRY _____ AGE _____ SEX _____ RACE (OPTIONAL) _____

PHONE _____ FAX _____

Completely fill in the appropriate circle for each question

	T F		T F		T F		T F		T F		T F
1	○ ○	31	○ ○	61	○ ○	91	○ ○	121	○ ○	151	○ ○
2	○ ○	32	○ ○	62	○ ○	92	○ ○	122	○ ○	152	○ ○
3	○ ○	33	○ ○	63	○ ○	93	○ ○	123	○ ○	153	○ ○
4	○ ○	34	○ ○	64	○ ○	94	○ ○	124	○ ○	154	○ ○
5	○ ○	35	○ ○	65	○ ○	95	○ ○	125	○ ○	155	○ ○
6	○ ○	36	○ ○	66	○ ○	96	○ ○	126	○ ○	156	○ ○
7	○ ○	37	○ ○	67	○ ○	97	○ ○	127	○ ○	157	○ ○
8	○ ○	38	○ ○	68	○ ○	98	○ ○	128	○ ○	158	○ ○
9	○ ○	39	○ ○	69	○ ○	99	○ ○	129	○ ○	159	○ ○
10	○ ○	40	○ ○	70	○ ○	100	○ ○	130	○ ○	160	○ ○
11	○ ○	41	○ ○	71	○ ○	101	○ ○	131	○ ○	161	○ ○
12	○ ○	42	○ ○	72	○ ○	102	○ ○	132	○ ○	162	○ ○
13	○ ○	43	○ ○	73	○ ○	103	○ ○	133	○ ○	163	○ ○
14	○ ○	44	○ ○	74	○ ○	104	○ ○	134	○ ○	164	○ ○
15	○ ○	45	○ ○	75	○ ○	105	○ ○	135	○ ○	165	○ ○
16	○ ○	46	○ ○	76	○ ○	106	○ ○	136	○ ○	166	○ ○
17	○ ○	47	○ ○	77	○ ○	107	○ ○	137	○ ○	167	○ ○
18	○ ○	48	○ ○	78	○ ○	108	○ ○	138	○ ○	168	○ ○
19	○ ○	49	○ ○	79	○ ○	109	○ ○	139	○ ○	169	○ ○
20	○ ○	50	○ ○	80	○ ○	110	○ ○	140	○ ○	170	○ ○
21	○ ○	51	○ ○	81	○ ○	111	○ ○	141	○ ○	171	○ ○
22	○ ○	52	○ ○	82	○ ○	112	○ ○	142	○ ○	172	○ ○
23	○ ○	53	○ ○	83	○ ○	113	○ ○	143	○ ○	173	○ ○
24	○ ○	54	○ ○	84	○ ○	114	○ ○	144	○ ○	174	○ ○
25	○ ○	55	○ ○	85	○ ○	115	○ ○	145	○ ○	175	○ ○
26	○ ○	56	○ ○	86	○ ○	116	○ ○	146	○ ○	176	○ ○
27	○ ○	57	○ ○	87	○ ○	117	○ ○	147	○ ○	177	○ ○
28	○ ○	58	○ ○	88	○ ○	118	○ ○	148	○ ○	178	○ ○
29	○ ○	59	○ ○	89	○ ○	119	○ ○	149	○ ○	179	○ ○
30	○ ○	60	○ ○	90	○ ○	120	○ ○	150	○ ○	180	○ ○

Special Discount Coupon

Please fill out and return the payment coupon below. This coupon
entitles readers to a $20 discount off the retail price of $59.95.
This special offer is available only with this coupon.
(Photocopies not accepted.)

Payment Method: Please include $39.95 (regular value $59.95; Michigan
residents add 6% sales tax), plus $4.55 for shipping and
handling.

☐ Personal check (Will be held three banking days before being released and
may be verified with a check clearing service. $10.00 penalty for returned
checks.)

☐ Money Order or Bank Check

☐ MasterCard (16 digits)

☐ VISA (13 or 16 digits)

_____

Customer Signature

_____

Card Account Number   Credit Card Expiration Date

Return this coupon, *with answer sheet only*, to: Robertson Institute, Ltd.,
Testing Division, 3555 Pierce St., Saginaw, MI 48604. You will receive your
personal enhancement plan in two to three weeks.